The Serpents Sting

Written By: Letitia Carter

Dedicated to:

To my children Ben and Rachel, My husband Gary, and all of those who have stuck by my side during this long road to recovery. This has been a long journey that has consumed over half my life, it has been a battle in which I will not give up nor give in until the day when I can hold my head up and my hands to the heavens and rejoice, When the battle has been won and the Serpent will be cast back into the shadows of darkness where it belongs. I give thanks to my Lord for giving me the strength to walk this life of temptations and endure the pain and suffering that has been cast upon me. I do not feel it was nothing less than a continued test of faith and a journey that would take me into the lives of many people who I only pray will see the light as I have and to know that God is there to walk each and every one of us to the finish line.

In Memory of my beloved sister and best friend Star

For my beautiful sister, her saving grace came in the form of death because the Lord knew this was ultimately the only way that she could be saved from the addiction and the disease of the Bacterial Meningitis which had left her paralyzed and relying on life support but it wasn't that she could not be saved from all of this, I knew my sister and I knew how hard she was fighting to survive and how desperately she wanted to beat this disease and all of the complications that had come along with having a traumatic brain injury. God knew that if he allowed her to survive that coming back home would only continue to drag her back into the pit with the Serpent and all the evil that lay in our small hometown, so he waited and gave her time to correct and make right the wrongs she had done in this life and then he placed her within his loving arms and took her home, to the paradise of Heaven where she can truly be free from the grasp of the Serpent.

For those who tried repeatedly, yet because of the relentless hold of addiction that took over the once vibrant existence died due to the Serpent's Sting, my sweet sister who could have under a completely different lifestyle, a better choice of friends and a deeper love for herself and the family, especially the two children who adored her e every waking moment especially her youngest child and constant caregiver Jess, because as long as Star was awake even if it meant being blown away on prescription pain killers it became good enough for that baby girl just in knowing that her Momma was breathing and still alive for yet another second, perhaps an hour, but as my sister's addiction rapidly escalated we all began to wonder if tomorrow would someday be that dreaded phone call when you don't want to even answer the phone anymore, when you see it is your sister's house or your Mother's number late at night for fear it will be that long dreaded news that my precious niece found her lifeless body only this time it was too late unlike all the other times when the emergency medical technicians had been able to revive her. That day came the morning after Thanksgiving 2010 when Star collapsed on the floor of our Mother's kitchen and that would be a morning that would change everyone's life forever.

The Serpents Sting

{The path we choose isn't always the path taken}
One family's story of addiction and recovery by the Grace
And love of Christ Our Lord

An Entire Families Life of Addiction

Looking up at the beautiful blue skies and green grass, I realize all that I have and all that I Had taken for granted for so many years during my path of self-destruction into the world of Prescription pain pill addiction I call the serpent's sting, though the journey was not only a slow treacherous path of pain and humiliation but also one of learning and establishing a relationship with God that only he can ever fully understand. I never thought a thing about the emblem or the serpents, I never thought about the destruction that can be handed down once we turn the outcome of our health over to someone other than Christ himself. I never realized just how powerful the evil forces which surround our inner beings can entangle our lives and cause a whirlwind of disasters which continually *create one failure after another until we have nowhere to go but a slow ride to a local mortuary or into the loving arms of our heavenly Father. We get to the point in our lives that we can sink no lower, we have already reached the gates of hell and being governed by the evil forces that have contaminated our bodies and destroyed our sense of reality, we sense that there is still that little hint of a compassionate entity lurking within us, calling out to us in a low almost unrecognizable voice and then you hear it, the voice of him ,Christ, the glorious sound of patience and he is whispering to you, come my child, I am here, do not fear for you are not alone, but you do not fully hear that voice while you are living in the worldly fashion that keeps the darkness lurking in anticipation just waiting to take over the body of that one more lost soul that doesn't have a clue that the journey they are about to take will be brutal, it will have no compassion for you and will not leave you alone for one minute until it has cast it's spell over your entire being .The day that I finally heard that splendid voice was the beginning of a battle that would end up lasting me a lifetime and Christ said so lovingly, In all the days that you have traveled that long and fearful journey you were not alone, for I was with you all the while. When you laid your head on tarnished ground, I gently held you up so that you wouldn't drown in the muck. When you were lost in the forest of the unthinkable excuses, I excused you for there was no one else there to help you take your next step forward. As you were crawling on a floor of splintered wood not knowing if the planks were filled with splinters standing erect and waiting to stab your very heart, I lifted you up and carried you toward the bed in which you laid your head to rest in soft comfort. There was never a time when I left you alone, oh child of mine, I have been with you all these days, just waiting for this* moment when you called out to me, asking to be saved by grace. To forgive you, you are forgiven. To lead you, I have laid the path for you to travel. I leave it up to you to choose the direction and as for my love, I have loved you all your days, even as you drifted away from me, my love was with you all the while. "Isaiah 48: 10 I have refined you, but not as silver is refined, I have refined you in the furnace of suffering" You may ask, why God would allow suffering to come to his children and to answer this is, God does test us through sufferings. Rather than continuing to complain we should seek God in faith for the strength to endure those sufferings for without the testing we will never know what we are truly capable of doing, and will not grow. Without the refining we will not become that much more pure and like Christ, he leads us to see that through facing our suffering and seeking him that God will refine us. God is like a loving parent who teaches and guides us even as we falter, stumble and fail. Peace and righteousness come to us when we listen and obey his Word. The harder my life became on the long and what has seemed like endless journey through my world of addiction the more I realized that I would never escaped the evil as long as I continued to ignore that voice and as the years continued to pass and as I continued to try to escape from the clutches of the enemies dark world I realized I would never be able to do it alone and that God was the only answer to my Saving Grace. When I began to let him take control of the illness and my diseased body the more I noticed that I was beginning to want less and less to do with any of the worldly choices brought on by dirty doctors and evil temptations from the serpent who knew my every weakness and use them all against me for the rest of my days to try to break the bond I was creating with my Lord. I saw that as long as I continue to give in to *my weakness no matter what it may be that the serpent will be in control and that as I continue to grow stronger in faith and seek God and continue to pray for strength and courage to overcome these afflictions God will continue to lift me up until I am free once and for all from the chains that have held me captive for a very large portion of my life. I share with all who will listen, about my family's journey in hopes that they too will hear and will seek to break free from these chains that have held us captive for what seems like an eternity and to know that they are not alone in the battle to overcome. The journey may be long but when the battle is finally won, you will experience the greatest sense of freedom you have ever known because you had the greatest power to carry you through when you chose the Holy Spirit as your strength, your guide, your courage, and your faith in God will you realize you were truly never alone when you stop to think about all the times you narrowly escaped death by overdose or maybe by being in the wrong place at the wrong time but you walked away unharmed when others were beaten, you will begin to see just how many times God protected and carried you out of harm's way because he believed in you even when you didn't believe in yourself and it wasn't time for your life to end because he has a greater life in store for you if you will follow his direction that he has made for each of us. He has created not one of us to be failures but to be his children and to live a good and prosperous life when we choose to do that which is our true journey in this life. May God be with all of us as we continue down the path that will lead us to Victory. Amen…….*

My days of addiction started in my teenage years. I was a child who suffered from severe allergies. I remember the ear, nose, and throat specialist telling my mother I would be better off living in a bubble. My worst allergies would just happen to be dust and smoke. In the springtime when everything was in full bloom my days were spent indoors away from the pollen. My eyes would swell shut, the cough was uncontrollable and I stayed miserable, until, the doctor prescribed me hydrocodone. This was a miracle drug. This opiate cured everything that ailed me. It stopped the cough, congestion and made me feel good. I honestly thought it was a miracle, but little did I know that this little prescription opiate which is used to treat a variety of ailments would end up leading me on a twenty four year journey, "The Serpents Sting", of drug addiction. I was slowly filled with the venom of this opiate pain killer, for nearly five years everything from the cough medicine to the pain medicine for my sinus headaches contained the drug, hydrocodone. This is a morphine derivative, used widely throughout the United States to alleviate pain. In those days the doctors forgot to tell you just how addictive this narcotic analgesic actually was and that it would end up being i abused by more than 200 million Americans as I write. It would take my doctor dying before I would begin to see that I was living in a world of addiction.

I didn't come from a broken home and my parents were not alcoholics and drug addicts, but just the opposite. I came from a Southern Baptist background, we went to Church on Sunday morning, Wednesday night, and Bible School every summer until I was just too old to go. I had two loving parent's, My Mother abused me for many years and always made a difference between me and my younger sister. It seemed I was the black sheep of the family.
.
We were not wealthy but we got everything we needed and a lot of what we wanted. My Father who had always Been a blue collar worker and the provider stepped back while Mom made the rules, she set the rules and if

you knew what was best you would abide by them respectfully. She was the disciplinarian and you would abide by the rules or face the consequences and all to often I questioned why I was being beaten. Mother apologized many years later for her behavior and the way she treated me but she never gave me an answer as to why it was me and not my sister or why she didn't do it to the both of us, It was not until my drug addiction manifested into a full blown life changing battle did I realize the true importance of family, friends and all the people you desperately need in this life, especially Christ but I also realized that all those years of my Mother's abuse had actually made me the person I am today. She did instill in me love for others, the importance of honesty, strength and she raised us to know God is always there no matter where you are whether it is in a mansion in Beverly Hills or a famine stricken apartment in the Bronx, He is there and when you allow him to be a part of your life and accept him as your Savior there is nothing you cannot do. My addiction is just another obstacle evil has placed in my way and what my Mother created was a daughter who would fight to survive and with God would win the battle.

In The Beginning

It all began with my Grandmother who suffered from severe depression, chronic heart problems, Breast cancer and one illness after another; it was easier back in those days to just pretend everything was alright. Her addiction was hidden by family rather than face the painstaking truth, the truth addiction due to years of using prescription pain killers for chronic pain due to her back pain, arthritis and so many health problems.

God above, my Grandfather, my Mother and the other seven brothers and five remaining sisters and with faith and many prayers an many miracles there would be only two more children fall victim to the cycle of opiate addiction and it was none other than the youngest daughter and the one woman who had refused to even take an aspirin for pain for fifty years until she was diagnosed with fibromyalgia at which time she began using opiate painkillers/hydrocodone, muscle relaxants, and anxiety medication better known as Xanax. When my sister became so ill before she later passed on December of 2011, Mom was taking so many of the Xanax that we were all afraid she might accidentally overdose and we watched her day and night for thirteen months until Star went home to Jesus; however though there was one thing the Lord knew he must do for Star before she went home with him. Christ gave Star the chance to be admitted to a Christian based community hospital for the last six months of her life. Upon admittance to that place the staff informed my Mother they had been very misinformed about my sister condition and that there was a very strong possibility she would make a significant improvement as time went on. The first hospital that had been over her care prior to being admitted to Jellico hospital was the University of Tennessee Trauma Unit. My sister was admitted and put into a drug induced coma immediately for her surgery. A team of over ten specialist including those from the Center for Disease Control. The doctors concluded she had contracted Bacterial Meningitis from snorting Roxycodone pain killers from a straw that had grown bacteria by being used repeatedly and Star had a severe Sinus infection that wasn't getting any better for several weeks and I was told she had gotten so weak after being hospitalized at two local hospitals one month apart and even admitted to I.C.U. but the attending physician there told her she could continue with the attending physicians kept asking my Mother if she had been using street drugs and of course the one time that she should have been had been seeing another specialist who she told mom completely honest but instead she chose to avoid the truth. It was not out of malice but love for her child that my Mother chose to pretend that her daughter who lay there fighting for her life was truly not an addict. Looking back at all of this now and at all of my family, I see that I came from a very dysfunctional place, there are so many secrets and skeletons lurking in everyone's closet, that if they ever break free, it will be like hell being unleash on Ivy Hollow.

When I left Tennessee, we moved everything we had in storage and left as if it had never existed. I was feeling well that day for I had went by my cousins and bought enough morphine for a few days but like every other time it would be gone way too early and I tried everything knew.. I lay in bed all week and fought the withdrawals with every ounce of strength I had in my body and please believe me after abusing a highly potent pain medication for 2 years and then stopping cold turkey, you could say I was definitely not myself. I have a pinched nerve from an injury years ago and it seemed that all of the pain was finding that area and attaching like a fly. I would lay in bed and toss and turn for hours, then I would sit in the hottest tubs of water I could tolerate without scalding myself. When the pain would finally get so severe that it felt like my insides were trying to rip out of my body and I would start convulsing so badly on the right side of my body that the first doctor thought I was having a severe epileptic seizure. Even though I was a very severe addict I wasn't one of those people who would hop from hospital to hospital looking for a fix, nor would I call every addict I knew to see if they might be willing to help me out. As bad as I hated this world I had come to now as an addict there was something that I loved more than any drug that would ever cross my lips or be injected into my body. I loved my Children! And my Lord above more than anything in this world and I was so tired of disappointing each one them, I thought about how God said I was created in his image, but I promise you this was not the image he was talking about. Every time I would stumble and fall right back to the dark and lonely world of addiction I knew deep within my heart that Christ would be there to catch me and hold me in his loving arms.[Psalms 11:4} After reading this psalm, but the Lord is in h s holy temple' he still rules from heaven. He watches everyone closely, examining every person on earth. I read about the unbelievers, the liars, the deceitful and the wicked that want to do nothing more than to hurt us when we are weak and helpless, remember these words when the foundations are shaking and you wish you could hide, remember that God is still in control. His power is not diminished by any turn of events. Nothing happens without his knowledge and permission. When you feel like running away----Run to God instead, he will restore justice and goodness on the earth in his good time.

Evil Lurked Around Every Corner

My Grandma would stay hidden away in her bedroom, in the dark for weeks at a time, locking her wooden bedroom door for fear that her alcoholic son, I'll call Chester-as well as child predator would not be able to Get into Her room as he had secretly done for many years until I discovered the truth as I entered my ~~early~~ Adult life to find out not only had my Grandma been prey to this poor excuse of life ~~this sickening excuse Of a man had victimized not only on Grandma~~ But his younger sister, cousins, nieces, and me at the age of nine years old on Christmas Eve 1972 when I fell Prey as he lay in bed drunk from his early Christmas ~~party as he had called it.~~ I walked to his room to tell him Merry Christmas ~~and~~ he took my hand and placed it on he had done was wrong I chose not to tell ~~Dad or~~ Mom ~~because~~ I knew Dad, would have killed him, so I decided to always stay away from him for my own safety and to watch out for my cousins so he didn't bother them. Finally to the Man who had molested her two daughters by beginning to prey on me and my sister in our early Teenage years by making us feel like we were so special. As we discussed it when we got older, he had promised us both the same things and when I thought I was protecting her by letting him touch me he was already molesting Star who was only fourteen years old and. little did I know he had rented a home on the lake and she told me stories that sickened me at the time, Star And her friends would cut school and go there and spend the day with Him so they could get wasted drinking booze ~~and smoking marijuana. He would give them~~ money to buy things like clothes, cassettes and make up To this day I find it hard to believe my Mom and I could have been so blind that I didn't see it then but I wasn't Living at home. I had a child of my own now and was living in my own apartment raising my son alone ~~E~~ven when my sister confronted her years later as she became a woman and the molestation Became a full blown affair my Mother turned her back on my sister and told her she was lying because She couldn't have him because he wanted her instead of my sister. He just lay there with that look of Victory and smiled to himself as my Mother broke my sister's spirit and when I should have spoken up That day to defend my sister I couldn't speak for no words would come from within as I listen to the way Mother spoke to the child that she loved more than life itself, and as I looked down at my own daughter Who was just a fragile two year old, I couldn't help but think that he might someday try to do the same ~~Thing~~ to my daughter I would never ~~knowingly~~ give him the chance to be alone with my baby ~~girl~~. I ask myself often ~~personal~~ tragedy's led to ~~the reason for~~ our Journey into the world of Addiction? I will not say that they are the reason ~~for it~~ but it seems that each of us were genetically open to become addicted to either drugs or alcohol and with all of the skeletons ~~That~~ my family tried so hard to keep hidden deep down, each ~~one~~ of us whether male or female just ~~tried~~ to hide the truth. ~~AS the seasons came and went we just made~~ ourselves oblivious to the fact That we had been violated as children ~~issues that should have been Addressed so many years ago. Children violated by The~~ perverted uncles, some Who acted out their hidden agendas When ~~They~~ thought they had found the perfect victim who would ~~stay~~ quiet and never tell anyone, But ~~never tell but~~ little did they Know I had already warned all my younger cousins ~~the girls both young and old~~ of the vicious cycle of their fondling ~~the~~ dangers that lay hidden way beneath ~~That seemingly~~ loving smile and that for their safety they should never be ~~alone~~ with these men because beneath that loving smile laid an evil dark man that would take away ~~their~~ childhood innocence by making them do things that were so very wrong. For the most part I have To say ~~that~~ all but a couple of My female cousins listened to me while the few that didn't were able to be ~~bribed~~ with money, alcohol and allowing them to drive at very young ages, usually nine or ten years old. My heart ached for them ~~then~~ just as it does today and I hope they have found peace within because I ~~know~~ they have to feel so violated now That they have grown into women with children of their own, I do know that none who Daughters of their own never took them around our uncle and even in his ~~death~~ not many cousins attended his funeral. We all seemed to have lost touch after childhood and when I did see them after all those years it seemed that we all still had more than just our uncles perverted ~~ways~~, We were ~~all~~ suffering from some form of Addiction, whether to prescription drugs or alcohol in ~~which~~ we used to numb the pain. In writing this to meet And I know they too have suffered many similar circumstances. In my journey, I found even the youngest addicts feel they have done too much wrong to ever be able to make Things right With the Lord. I remember the words I once read in scripture, "We are all sinners and fall short of the Glory of God" BUT "through our repentance and acceptance of our Savior Jesus Christ who died on the Cross so that we could be saved, means just that... When we accept Jesus into our hearts and we ask Him for forgiveness for the sins we have committed, "We Are forgiven!" Unlike those of us who have Lied, cheated, stolen, killed or whatever the case may be, we can be forgiven if we truly want it and With that comes the promise of Eternal Life in The Kingdom of Heaven with God Almighty! AMEN....

Fighting the Evil All throughout Our lives

I was a sickly child, mother said at the age of 14 months I became very anemic and decided I was just too tired to walk anymore. This began my repeated trips to the pediatrician. It seemed like I would no sooner get well from one sickness until another would strike. The doctors did repeated testing but could find nothing wrong. At the age of nine I was to begin throwing large amounts of blood from my kidneys. I gained over twenty pounds of unexplainable fluid and I looked like a balloon ready to pop. After being admitted to two hospitals I was eventually diagnosed with nephritis a kidney disease that was said to have manifested from an untreated strep infection and it was hard for anyone to believe since mom took us to the doctor if we sneezed. After being on bed rest for almost a year, I was finally allowed to go back to school and live a somewhat normal life, but no hard jumping, no over exertion and no hard licks to the kidneys. I didn't feel very normal. I was given liquid valium because due to my kidneys and over active bladder I was not always able to control my urinating. The doctor said this would help as well as take care of my anxiety. It seemed I had also been diagnosed with what they called high anxiety back in the day. That begin the lifelong use of anti-anxiety medication such as valium and later on Xanax but I never seemed to have a problem with addiction when it came to using those medications. I would go for months without them until the anxiety would come back but I never used them every day of my life, they were the one drug I actually took as prescribed.

    At the age of ten, I came down with the most severe case of chicken pox my pediatrician had ever seen. I remember it so well. It was Easter Sunday and while sitting at church I noticed a sore on the side of my face that itched terribly. I thought nothing of it and by the time I got home from church they were spreading My mom called the doctor as usual and he said it was fall sores I have no idea to this day what that was suppose too mean.} Back when I was a child it seemed like the doctors would make up names for ailments they couldn't diagnose. The next morning I awoke to have oozing sores all over my body, even in my mouth. My eyes were swollen shut and I was in misery. Chicken pox was the problem. Once again I was laid up at home. This lasted for a little over a month and I was released to go back to school.

At the age of eleven I awoke the second week of sixth grade to look in the mirror and see the right side of my face swollen twice the size it should have been. I was diagnosed once again with one of the worst cases of the mumps and once again I was taken out of school on medical leave. It seemed as though I was never going to get to go to school like a normal kid. The seventh and eighth grade was good. I thought I was really out of the woods. I had continuous stomach aches, but after doctor visits, hospital stays and test, I was just diagnosed with a nervous stomach, whatever that meant. I also had a thyroid disorder which I had been treated for since the age of ten, this was said to have also been one of the reasons for my anxiety, the worst was the leg pain that would wake me at night screaming in agony and begging momma to make it stop. I would be hospitalized and series of tests later there would be a diagnosis of a nervous stomach and growing pains.

My freshman year of high school was great, new school, new friends, and boom! Mono nucleosis . Apparently I had caught it from a water fountain at school. Once again I was put on medical leave from school. I was admitted into the hospital with a 105 degree temperature, isolated from everyone except my mother who wore a mask, but never left my side. I remember being so sick that I could barely open my eyes. My mom had to leave the hospital due to my little sister being diagnosed with a brain infection. She too was there in the same hospital in quarantine and we didn't know whether she would make it. I didn't know at the time how my parents made it through all the traumatic experiences with me and now with my little sister. God was the answer then even if I may have not fully understood when I was younger I still remember hearing the ministers pray for me and my sister. I remember my mom crying and my dad holding her in the corner of my hospital room. My Mother was the strongest woman I have ever known. She never slept, she was with us day and night and I just thought she was an angel. She never got sick, she always made you feel better and she definitely made you feel safe, she was the greatest. After about a week I got to go home from the hospital and a few days later my sister would be cleared and released from isolation. She recovered rather quickly; however, I wasn't so lucky. For six months I was put on bed rest and once again I was home schooled and kept from my peers. My life was doomed and I wandered if I was ever going to get to live a normal life.

    You are probably wondering what this has to do with my addiction. I wondered that myself as I was looking back on my life and trying to find out where my life took a turn into the direction of drugs. Every therapist I have seen has explained to me it wasn't a choice but due to the extreme amount of physical illness, surgeries, and years of continuous health problems actually led to what they prefer to call dependence because I wasn't using the drugs to get high but to help the symptoms and pain that came with everything. I didn't remember standing up in my third grade class and giving an oral report on "When I grow up I want to be a drug addict." I didn't remember in all my stays in the hospital any nurses or doctors saying to me or my parents, we are sorry to inform you, but, your child has been diagnosed with addiction, a disease caused by many years of having to use the opiate pain killers we *have given to her. I spent many years trying to piece together how my life could have gotten so screwed up, so bad, so fast. It wasn't fast, just the opposite. From the time we are created, evil forces lie in waiting around us, waiting for that perfect moment in which to attack. They begin by breaking us down. Little by little, they take our strength and turn it into our weakness. If we are weak and sickly children then the evil forces play on that just as they did with me. For so many years they broke me little by little. I was diagnosed with one sickness after another. With each sickness came medication, medication that would make my body slowly become dependent, I would slowly become dependent on those drugs in order to function in what I would think to be a normal way of life.*

At the age of sixteen the principal of the high school in which I had attended on a pretty much part-time basis informed my parents that it would be in my best interest to let me go ahead and drop school and pick up my diploma with a GED. This being because once again I would be being admitted to the hospital for surgery on my bladder and then immediately following that I would be having surgery on my foot from an accident a couple of years earlier. Once again I would be laid up at home, home bound teaching was just another way of saying I was getting at least a little bit of an education, because most of the time the teacher couldn't come to the house because I was contagious, and- neither of my parents had made it even into high school, so they wouldn't be able to help me in any of my classes.

In October of 1979 I withdrew from school. I was devastated that I would not be graduating the following summer with my graduating class of 1980, but according to everyone, this was for the best. I was behind in the credits I needed to graduate anyway, so I could take the aptitude test, get my GED and go to college just like everyone else. Apparently when the evil that has laid in waiting for you most of your life sees the chance to grab hold, it strikes full force. I began having such horrific sinus infections and headaches that I couldn't stand to be in the same room with the people I loved. The physician began prescribing me the hydrocodone pain killers. These were the miracle drugs that began my journey into the most horrific years of my life.

At the age of twenty three I had been taking the pain medicine for over seven years. With sometime off in between. I had my first child, a son, at the age of twenty, and during that time I never took anything not even a Tylenol. God was watching over me then because during my pregnancy I never once experienced any problems with my allergies or had any of the headaches like before. He was there with me to protect my unborn child from the dangers of the drugs, while I was pregnant I never once thought about those pain killers but- after his birth the symptoms came right back. ~~at the time I really didn't know that I was really an addict either,~~ I believe I began to see the ~~true~~ addiction ~~began~~ three years later when my ear, nose and throat specialist died suddenly, leaving me without the medication that I had practically made a daily regimen just as if it were a vitamin. At first I had no idea what was going on, all that I knew was I was so sick, I was so congested, I was hurting all over, my legs were in excruciating pain and the sweats were terrible, I thought I had the flu; however when I went to my new doctor who prescribed me the same medications as before, the flu was gone in less than an hour. This was truly a miracle pill. It even cured the flu. I was so unaware of addiction to prescription medications that I truly did not know that I was *suffering from addiction or that what I had just identified as the flu was actually withdrawals from the miracle pill that had become a daily regimen in my life. This would begin my journey into The Serpents Sting.*

Once I realized that I had a problem with the prescription pain killers I decide that I would seek treatment so I made an appointment with the local behavioral health clinic and went over my options with a counselor. He decided my best option for treatment would be to check into an inpatient treatment facility, so he made the calls and set up a check in -time. I was to go home and make arrangements for my son and talk to my family and three days later check in for treatment.

The big mistake was confronting my mother about my disease. Mom was a little more than upset , she was furious. I'll never forget those words as long as I live, "I didn't raise a weak ass to be a daughter of mine." Her reply cut into my soul like that of a triple edge sword and as those words cut into my heart a piece of me agreed. Her next response was, " you are not going to embarrass me in front of the whole community." This was a no win situation for me, now not only was I feeling like a failure as a daughter but as a mother also. I couldn't leave my son for a whole month. It would be a week before I would get to see him once I checked into the facility and then once a week for a month. So I decided to do it alone. I was a strong woman and I could do this, it couldn't be that hard. For the next week I lay in bed once again with that darn flu, only this time it seem to be a lot worse than the last time. This time I knew it was actually the withdrawal symptoms from the drugs. I ran a fever, chills, sweats, body aches, and somewhere in there had a few minor breakdowns. I prayed, and I prayed for God to raise me up from the grasp of this affliction. On the third day, I awoke to find that most of the symptoms had vanished. Thank you God I replied as I realized it wasn't taking a great deal of effort to climb out of bed. Never again I told myself that day as I looked at my little boy sitting there on the bed beside me, never again will I put him through this I whispered. For seventy two hours he had stayed there beside me as I fought to make it through the effects of the withdrawals, him thinking I truly had the flu. He was such a precious, and innocent three year old child who deserved nothing more than to be loved and to be happy. It was the summer of 1986, and a new beginning for me and my family.

God works within us all throughout our lives in ways we do not always understand. And sometimes bad things happen to us not to hurt us but sometimes they are used as tools of learning and preparing us for things to come later on in life. I was about to embark in a journey of darkness, emptiness, sadness, loneliness and many times a life of sheer torture, all in which would turn out to bring me closer to God than I have ever been before, more understanding, stronger, a woman of godly discipline and respect, and someone who knows all too well that this world and all that are in it is too much for us to go it alone. We cannot create a foundation of principals and self =worth without accepting Christ into our life. There is no happiness and no sense of accomplishment without abiding by the word of Christ and following the rules he has set for us as we travel on this earthly journey. When we fall by the way or off the path that Christ has laid out for us we will run into many obstacles and temptations that will forever try to keep us from finding our way back to the straight and righteous direction in which we are meant to travel. There is much to be done during our short stay here on earth. There are millions and millions of people, many who are lost and in need of being introduced to Christ. It is our destiny to help in spreading the word throughout the world. To join together as children of God and help in introducing those lost to Jesus, to Christianity, to let them know that they too can have their name placed into the Book of Life, to live eternally with the Father. Oh! What a glorious day that will be. When there is no more sorrow, no more sin, but peace and happiness and good will toward men forever and ever, Amen..

It was 1992 all was good, my son and I were living in a little house in the country that my Grandfather had built back after the depression. I had always wanted to live there just for the simple fact that papaw had built it. Things were going good. I was pregnant with my second child, another little miracle since all odds had been against me to ever have children. It was one of those unbelievably hot summers, humid, sticky, just down right miserable but it was still a great summer.

Summer came and went, as did Christmas and another new year rolled around. 1993, this was going to be a great one, on January 15th I gave birth to a beautiful baby girl and on my son's tenth birthday not only did he get all of his much wanted army gear but a brand new baby sister, which he would have probably preferred to have left at the hospital. All kidding aside he was a wonderful brother. After the birth of my daughter it was the recommendation of the doctors that I have no more children due to the stress it was causing my kidneys. So I scheduled a surgery for prevention of it ever happening again. Of course they had to prescribe the same pain killers that I had so desperately fought to stay away from for so long. I figured that since it had been such a long time since I had taken them that they wouldn't hurt me to use them for a few days after my surgery. Don't ever believe that you will never go back. To this day I wish I had never put that first pill into my mouth that day. I didn't go back into a full blown addiction, oh that wouldn't happen for a few more years down the road. I became a dabbler, I took them when I was prescribed them from the doctors, but I never abused them so I thought I was alright. In 1997 something snapped, I don't really know if it was the fact that I married a man who went to jail for a year two months after our marriage, I don't know if it was because I lost my vehicles and had nothing to drive, I don't know if it was the fact that we were going to lose our home. I think that everything just became too much for me to handle and ~~as usual the~~ pills ~~were~~ my escape from reality. While my husband was incarcerated I began using the pain killers to just plain feel better. Due to depression, I stayed tired all the time, so the pills gave me energy. I didn't have a car or a way to get around, so the pills made it easier to bare. I felt so helpless ~~was just plain lonely~~, so the pills made me ~~think I felt~~ better, oh what a mistake that was. By the time my husband was released from jail I was right back to my previous full blown addiction that I had been free from since 1993. The day he called me to tell me he was coming home I really didn't care because first off, I was out of pain killers and second how could I be happy when my son had just buried his best friend at the age of 16 after a car wreck in which by the grace of God he had not been a passenger that night because the boy's had been running late and had decided to pick Ben up after they returned from Newport to pick up a motorcycle. We had just returned from the funeral service when I received the call that I could pick my husband up from the county jail. How could I truly be happy when my world had fell apart, I had been stranded in this house for almost a year, never leaving unless my Dad came and picked me up to *go to the store or to go to his house for a while to visit. This man had left me to handle everything alone for all that time and never apologized once for all he had put me and my children through; however he called daily begging me for over ten months to do something to get him out of jail. A week after his release from jail and after I had taken every penny I had to pay what bills I could including partial rent we were served an eviction notice and that just threw me further into my depression not knowing how we were going to get out of this situation, but once again God pulled us through and we were given yet another chance to piece our lives back together. I didn't realize at that time I had married a man who I would discover to be one of the most irresponsible people I had ever met. I should have seen and gotten out of the marriage then but due to my addiction and fear that I couldn't make it on my own which I had been doing for years before I met him, working and raising my children alone because I didn't want to get married or be tied down to any man I made the mistake of saying I do to this man when he came into my life through my son after his father's death in 1997. My son loved him and thought he was the greatest and wanting nothing more than to make my son happy I made the mistake of marrying him before really getting to know and what a deceiver he truly was. I stayed in this marriage not out of love but my Christian belief that marriage vows are sacred. I would found out as the years continued to bring me and my children one form of grief after another and as I was emotionally abused to the point of being just a broken body of a once strong and beautiful woman now an addict without a job, without a car, a made prisoner in my own home by a man who cared nothing for anyone but himself. I would learn as the years passed that he would feed off of my addiction by keeping me on the medication in order to keep me from leaving him, which would cause unbearable pain for me and my children to the point that my son would go into his own world of depression and addiction and yet God was there to bring forth a mentor into my daughter's life who would help her to grow in faith and keep her in close contact with the church and the Christian community that would lead her to have a relationship with God that would grow and blossom into such a spiritual blessing that would lead her into a world of godliness and away from home to a life of college, church, leadership abilities and leading others to seek Christ. God saved her from falling into the web of failure and addiction by leading her out of harm's way and I praise he each day for all he has done for my precious daughter. I prayed that someway, somehow that he would also help my son to also find his way out of the darkness that had engulfed his life because I felt so guilty for so much that had caused his misfortune due to my failing marriage and the stagnant relationship that came to be with him and my husband who wanted nothing more than to break my family because as I would later learn he was such a broken man himself. He was a closet addict, alcoholic and would over a fifteen year marriage never admit to his mistakes but blame someone else for all of his Misfortunes. As my life continued to fall apart my addiction continued to escalate until I was out of control but yet Inside I was screaming to be set free. It was a pain I would never wish upon anyone.*

The years passed by and the seasons came and went. I really don't know if the summers were hot or if the winters were cold because my brain had become reliant on the pills in a way only an addict could understand. I didn't pay much attention to anything except the drugs. They had become my best friend, my true love, my companion. Without them I was nothing but a-bed ridden cripple, unable to function in society. I wasn't able to be a mother, a daughter, wife, friend or anything else. My life had been taken away by a little blue, white, pink, whatever color the pill of the day may have been. I went to stronger and stronger milligrams and more dangerous pills. From 1998 until 2000 I began using oxycontin 80mg. and morphine. These drugs are what society calls, a monkey on your back. It wasn't like any monkey I had ever seen smiling playfully from behind the mesh wire of the local zoo. It was as though a vicious beast had ripped from within my body ripping my flesh and leaving my insides lying on the floor in a puddle of fluids unknown to man. I had never been so sick .I was so weak that I could barely crawl to the bathroom and too weak to hold my head up to throw up. The withdrawals from these drugs were so horrific that I could do nothing but lie in bed and fight for survival, to make it through the night in hopes of a brighter tomorrow. I finally beat it once again, once again I was living the good life, the sober life, but something just wasn't right. Something was still missing and I just couldn't put my finger on it. The time has come, he said, "The Kingdom of God is near. I knew [Mark-1:14] God was calling, but I wasn't listening, or maybe I just didn't feel like I was deserving of him at this point in my life. I had done nothing but disappoint him once again.

In the summer of 2001 my dear, dear father was diagnosed with cancer. We as a family were devastated. The man we had always looked up to had been diagnosed with terminal lung cancer. He was given radiation treatments to try to slow the cancer down but it didn't work. My family decided that he should live with me and my family. They didn't ask me what I wanted; I just came home from work to find my mom sitting with my dad on my carport

said no but my addiction was right there leading me on and my father believed in me more than anything. He had always came to me when he needed legal advice, paperwork, someone to help him keep his finances in order and I loved him with all my heart, but, Daddy was my enabler, he was always there to give me his pain meds to get my money so I wouldn't go out and spend it on the streets that way when I needed it he would always have it to give back. I knew that I was entering dangerous territory but I would not turn my back on the man who had raised me creeping out of every crook and cranny. He was prescribed Lora tab, morphine liquid, morphine pills, it was an addict's paradise, but I wasn't at all happy because I had been struggling with sobriety for the past several weeks at the time daddy found out about his cancer I told myself that I was going to beat this demon. For once in my life I was going to be the strong one. I would take care of my daddy and be the good daughter, wife and mother of my children, I would not let the evil control my life anymore.

I couldn't have been more wrong, as dad got worse, he didn't sleep and if he did, he wanted me to be there lying by his side. I would hold him like he was a little child and pull him close to comfort him. Daddy may have been sixty eight years old, but he was as spoiled as a three year old toddler. What my Grandmother hadn't done to ruin him, my mom and stepmother had continued through the years, and now all he had was me, my kid's and my husband. Every night I would lie down in my bedroom with my husband and every night about an hour later, dad would call out to me or start to beat on the walls. I began to wear down and I was exhausted both physically and emotionally. I began to have a lot of back pain and horrific migraine headaches. One morning I awoke to a pain in my head so furious that it blinded me. My dad was calling for me in one room, and my daughter was calling in the other. On the window sill of my room sat a bottle of liquid morphine. I fought it for hours and then I gave in, if this medication could ease the pain of the cancer eating away at my dad's insides, it would help my head. That was the true beginning of my eighteen month nightmare, the morphine would- release me from the pain but it ~~would turn out to be my~~ release from total reality. My dad was dying and I was falling deeper and deeper into The Serpents Sting.

For eighteen months I lived and breathed pain killers. They had become my release from the reality that I was losing my dad,-something that I didn't want to accept, I didn't even want to think about it. I found that if I took enough of the pills, the pain from it all would just disappear. Daddy's condition continued to deteriorate and with that my addiction grew, I was consuming liquid morphine, morphine pills, anything that could make me forget the devastating effects my daddy's pending death was having on me. I was able to put on a face of pure false feelings in order to care for my dad as if I were an expert in the field of cancer, but the truth was I would set in the bedroom with my daddy, my feet dangling off the bed as they use to when I was a little girl and he and I would sit and talk about our days and how we spent them. We would talk about the cancer and he would ask me what I thought, did I think chemo was a good ideal since the radiation hadn't worked. It was a question I didn't know the answer to so I told him, daddy you do what feels right in your heart. I already knew that he would try the chemotherapy because more than anything my dad wasn't ready to die, he wanted to live, for me, my sister, but for his baby girls, his granddaughters and grandsons daddy just wasn't ready to go. I watched him daily as he sat there on his bed, he would hold his fragile little head in his hands as if thinking the deepest of thoughts, I knew they were the thoughts of death, they were thoughts of fear, of being alone, of leaving all those he loved so desperately. Together dad and

I would pray, asking God to spare his life and we prayed for God to give him the chance to be the man that he had once been when he was married to my mother. It was so sad to sit and watch how my daddy's face would light up when my mother walked into room. It was the look of the young football jock his junior year before homecoming, contemplating on asking that beautiful girl to the homecoming dance. How was it possible that my dad could still be as gitty as he was thirty eight years before when he had married mom. My mom knew had daddy felt so she would come and visit and bring those smiles of happiness to my daddy but she would have to walk away. I really wished she could have at least gave him a little more reason to fight for his life and maybe he could have beat it, because as the time went on dad slowly began to lose all will to live. I became so sick from my addiction that I checked myself into the local hospital for treatment and had my daddy checked in the next day We were 8 rooms apart and due to my guilt from my addiction I couldn't face my daddy, God brought him to my room one day and as he entered I fell apart, he held me close and whispered with what voice he had left. My precious little one, I love you know matter what, you have fallen victim to life's sinful temptations, you are not alone my little princess, for what I did in life by living and choosing also to follow those temptations I have ended up here. I smoked cigarettes for 40 years knowing the consequences that could happen if I didn't stop. I am here because I put myself here, you my child are here because you don't want this life and you are trying by the Grace of God, the Holy one, to conquer this affliction. It will not be easy and may times you may fail but the day will come my child when the Holy Spirit will raise you up and you will win the battle and then you will tell the story in which many will need to know, so that they too may live. Not long after that my dad past away, it was a warm spring night and I went to see him that one last time, I held him close and rocked him in my arms as he lay his head softly upon my shoulder as I sang to him Jesus loves me, A few hours later he was gone, but it is eight years later and all that my daddy told me that day was as if he were speaking of a premonition. Daddy died in April of 2002, I was taking the painkillers, but it was different, I was taking them only to survive, so I wouldn't be sick with the severe withdrawals so I took just enough of the medication to keep from getting sick. I didn't know what else to do except pray. I had tried re-habs, detox centers, cold turkey at home, everything and nothing worked. I knew it would be by the Grace of God that I would stop using these drugs. For twenty years I had been able to hide my addiction, but with my dad's illness and my extensive abuse of the pain killers it became impossible to hide it anymore. My daughter who was then eight only knew that mommy felt bad a lot. As long as I had the drugs, I was super mom, super wife, and just plain old super woman without the cape of course. As with every good feeling comes the feeling of utter pain and torture. It is an inevitable process with drug addiction. The feel good was gone, I was sad and lonely, and I felt like everyone I loved had given up on me, even my children. It wasn't until later on that I realized just how much pain I had caused my precious baby girl. She sat there at the age of 9 and told me of the many sleepless nights in which she had laid and cried herself to sleep while praying that I would live to see morning or in her eyes that I would just live. She told me how lonely it would be to be without her mother, how lost she would be not having me to do the little things like brush her hair before school in the mornings or to read her favorite book as she laid her beautiful little head on my shoulder at night. This was more than I could bear. It was at that moment when I looked into those beautiful, tear filled eyes that I made a promise not only to her but to myself that I would conquer this addiction. I didn't know how and I didn't know exactly when but in my heart I knew the serpent that had wrapped me within its powerful grip for all those years would release me in the name of God Almighty. I knew at that moment I would one day be free of this affliction.

Leaving It All Behind

In October of 2002 God graced my family by giving us the opportunity to move out of our hometown to South Carolina. My husband had gotten a contract job at the Charleston Air Force Base. This was as he said God's way of getting me away from the drugs and the access which I had to the drugs. We put everything we had into a storage unit and drove our old beat up truck to South Carolina. I wasn't happy, not by any means, I was terrified. We had brought enough medication to do me for a week and then it would be gone. Within two days the morphine was gone and I was sick, so sick that I had to crawl from the bed to the bathroom. My husband and son would leave for work and my daughter would catch the bus to school and I would lie there and scream and pray to God for him to please take the pain from my body. I had never hurt so severely in my life. I felt as though someone had attached *my legs to a vise and was slowly ripping me apart limb by limb. My fever was extremely high, for days I ran a fever of 103 and I was delirious. I prayed for God to take me, to let me die, for death would be so inviting for me at this point in my life. The first two months we would travel back to Tennessee every weekend to buy enough pills for a couple of days of relief for me, then to my astonishment my husband looked at me one day and said, enough is enough, you are one of the strongest women I have ever met, you were the best Mother a child could ever ask for. The evil temptation of drug addiction has taken the woman that I fell in love with and turned her into a selfish, unlikable creature that is slowly losing her family. These words coming from the man who had made sure he had morphine for my use but little did I know he too had fallen into the grasp of the addiction himself to ease his back pain. I told myself all his cruelty had been due to his fighting his own demons and that if we could break the cycle things would get better. I began to cry and at that point I knew that after my son had left and went back to Tennessee, my daughter stayed sad and depressed because I was living in bed hidden under the covers, moaning as that of a person dying from a terminal illness. I finally realized I had to stop all of it. On January 21,2003 I stopped everything. It was the sickest I had ever been in my life but I was determined to beat this disease, and I would with the help of my family and my God above. For three months I lay in bed in such pain and agony that sometimes death would have been a joyous occasion. I prayed to God continuously, to carry me through the battle, to lift me* up and cast out the evil that had afflicted my once faithful body. I knew that with God's love and my faith that I could beat this death sentence Satan had issued upon me. God was my strength, my breath and my reason for surviving, for recovering from an all too often killer," accidental drug overdose is becoming one of the number one killers of Americans today. I did not want to be one of those fatalities, I wanted to live.

My Family, My Lord, My Angels, My Saving Grace

My daughter was the one who was my little angel, one of the two earthly gifts God had blessed me with, my children wanted or ask for nothing more than to have the mother who had always been there for them-before the drugs had taken their control over my daily life's choices. When you are faced with the horrible fact that you are an addict, the drugs come first and fore most in your life, before your children, before your spouse, before your health, but most of all they come before your Lord and Savior, and even though you will argue with that it is a fact the drugs come before everything because without them you can no longer think rationally or function in society without them, so as bad as it hurt me to admit it there was no denying it. The one whom I was begging daily to release me from this drug infested body, the one who had blessed me with my life, the one who had blessed me with two beautiful children, the one who continued all these years to stand beside me, to carry me when I could no longer walk on my own two feet, I had forgotten him, not forgotten, but I had pushed him to the back of my mind *until the moment came and the bottom had fallen out of my life, only then did I call out for him. I prayed, Dear Father in Heaven how I need you, I am broken, my life is in shambles and I know not where to turn. I have been bad, I have let all that is unjust and unholy become the decision makers of my life. I am at your mercy Lord, for even as I traveled the journey of the serpent I knew Lord that you were waiting, waiting for your wayward drifting child to come home. I had fallen and drifted so far off of the path of righteousness that I truly was frightened that my Father in Heaven was so ashamed and angry with me that he would not hear my cries for help. As I lay there and prayed I then saw a vision. There was a door, and I stood at the entrance knocking, the door opened and there stood a manly form before me. I fell to my knees and began to cry uncontrollably, asking, Father I have been so shamed and I have disappointed you so. I have done things and traveled into such evil places that no man should ever have to take part in. The evil temptations that were set before me in my time of weakness was cruel and that of a liar yet I was too sickened to turn away from his gripping power until now. I was so frightened that he would close the door and tell me to leave his door at once to never return, yet instead he stood there without stretched arms and welcomed me into them saying, do not cry my child from that of shame but rejoice in love and know that all the time while you were traveling down your path of self- destruction, I was there, I never left your side, when you were in danger I kept you safe and when you needed to breathe the air of life I gave that breath back to you for* your time is not yet up. Your purpose of this life has not yet been fulfilled. Know that My love for you is forever and eternal, and even in times of sin it is still unconditional. Now that you have ended the destructive journey in which evil led you astray, take heed. The time is now that you speak of your experience, of your life and the choices in which everyone is given. We all have the choice to do either that which is good or that which is unholy. You did not travel the journey of the serpent by saying I chose to follow that which is evil, you were led by the power of deception and betrayal and many will be led to follow in that same journey as this earthly life continues. Use your experience and the wisdom placed upon during your travels through the dark side of humanity as a tool for teaching all that you encounter that they may not have to experience the turmoil of evil destruction in their lives, that through your experience you can open their eyes to see what will come to them if they also choose to follow that same path. Hold nothing back as you express your pain and anguish during your trials and tribulations in hopes that they may truly hear all that you have to say. Let all who listen know that even to take the smallest taste of that which is unholy and unclean can lead them into unfamiliar territory of evil companions who will be lying in waiting to devour their souls. Help all people both young and old that they may know that through faith and all that is good, that which is evil shall be destroyed and lifted up and away from the righteous. Through you my child, life has a special meaning, you are the one who will speak, the story teller of a life saved by grace, a child of God who by *believing in the power of healing by faith was given a life of new in hopes of introducing the Lord and Savior to all who will be Blessed by her words of spiritual bonding with Christ.*

My husband who loved me more than I ever deserved, my son who is happy to have the mom back he had always known would come back. The 18 months in which I fought my battle with morphine made it very clear that for me it was the most horrific experience I have ever endured. It was nine months before I could truly say I didn't want or need that drug anymore. That I could survive sober which is the greatest high I have ever known. In becoming sober, it was as if I had been reborn. I truly had to learn to live all over again. As I became more sober I realized I had become a lot older, a lot wiser and so thankful for all that I had accomplished and though I knew I still had a very long journey ahead of me I was so grateful for, "My Lord and my family who stood beside me through it all." More than anything in this world or the universe I am so grateful to my Lord and Savior Jesus Christ for never giving up on me, his lost sheep who wandered away from the flock. As Jesus said, "do not worry about your life, what you will eat, or you're your body, what will you wear, whom of you by worrying can add a single hour to your life? Since you cannot do this little thing, why worry about the rest? Do not be afraid little flock, for your Father has been pleased to give you the Kingdom. Sell your possessions and give to the poor. For where your treasure is, there your heart shall be also. '[Luke 27:34}

'Never Feel that you are not worthy in God's eyes, for the righteousness from God through faith in Jesus Christ to all who believe. There is no difference for all have fallen short of the glory of God and are justified freely by His grace through the redemption that came by Christ Jesus. '[Romans 3 22:26]

How Did It All Affect My Children

In the many days of my addiction, my precious daughter watched and listened, we talked about how I thought I had ended up in the situation and I explained it was a series of events that just kept leading me down the wrong path. I explained to her that I never intended to become an addict. Today my daughter is a 20 year old young woman who just finished her sophomore year in college and will begin the Nursing Program this fall. Rachel an avid member of the local church and she devoted her life to Christ at the early age of eleven. She is a youth leader and prayer leader, she is a volunteer, and she attends bible study group sessions weekly. My addiction saved my daughter's life. In all the bad and evil that she saw take part in my life, she found that above all else when it came down to the final decision to survive and live that my life was given to God utterly and completely. The summer of 2011 Rachel packed up all of her belonging and was off for college nine hours away to The University of Northern Alabama, she was on the adventure of a lifetime and even though I cried hysterically, I knew it was all for the best, I just wanted to save her from the continuing self ,destructive path she had been watched so many of her family members travel down for so very long and I wanted her to have a chance to succeed in life and to be happy and not have to wonder daily if me or her brother would be high, as I would try to explain to her, honey I promise you I am not high but just trying to survive and that was honestly the case, I didn't want to take any of the medication anymore, but the pain that had crept up on my body from a variety of injuries, ailments and being diagnosed with severe Arthritis and Fibromyalgia caused me to have to take the pills just to have some quality of life other than spending my days in bed because the pain was too severe to get up or move I know I caused her more grief than she ever deserved but someday I truly hope she understands it was not me but the addiction that had taken over my very being. I prayed God would protect her and keep her safe as she ventured out into the world alone but I knew God was with her every step of the way.

My dear, sweet son, who even though he was disgusted by the drugs fell victim himself and had also fought his own world of addiction since his early teenage years. He too never stood up in class and said when I grow up I too want to be a drug addict. When we get lost as children and begin to experiment with drugs we do not understand the consequences of prolonged us or the possibility of addiction for we believe we are invincible and that nothing can hurt us, not realizing until we are face down in the gutter of addiction, stealing, fighting, lying and anything we have to do to score that next high that we have been faced with a force way too strong for us to conquer on our own. Too many times the ultimate high is death. The addict continues to chase the dragon looking for that ultimate high that inevitably leads to death. Some addicts choose to die because the pain of addiction and the hurt of disappointment to their parents and loved ones becomes too much for them to handle, and they choose at the time what seems to be the only way out, not realizing that their parents would have given anything if they had just called or came to them and told them of their heartbreaking situation. I knew of my son's addiction and I worried continuously about his safety and whether or not he would die due to his own horrid love affair with some very potent and lethal drugs such as ecstasy, acid, pain killers, heroine, crack cocaine and powder cocaine. There were days when he would do ecstasy that I would sit and watch him sweat as that of a person on their death bed as they begin to lose their bodily fluids. His jaws would begin to constrict and he would turn so pale and cold. He thought that was the greatest high and would tell me how great it felt not realizing that he was on the brink of death for that is the ultimate high. Many nights I drove throughout the night searching for him because I did not know whether I would find him alive or dead and the times that he was arrested and taken to jail I would find myself so relieved for I knew he was still breathing. It didn't matter that I was an addict it was something that I never wished upon my children but just the opposite. I prayed that God would save them from that disease, from that evil journey that would cause them to make very poor choices and lead them on a path of destruction. My son is now thirty and still fighting with his addiction to opiates. Like me he too has been in and out treatment at a local methadone facility and he says that he this time he wanted to do it right. This was his second time of going this route of treatment and the professionals say that the program takes approximately six years to complete successfully. He also suffers from ADHD and bipolar disorder as well as depression which he is now currently being treated for and I prayed that God would show him the way because he could not succeed if he didn't work to correct all of the problem not just the physical effects but also the emotional instability . In the past ten years I have watched his addiction take from him so many things in his young life. He has two beautiful children, a little girl who just turned six whom he hasn't seen in almost two years and a nine year old son he hasn't seen sense he was six months old and it is all due to his addiction to drugs. I know this has to hurt him so badly because I know the man my son can be and I know the kind of father he will be if he can just get his life in order and in balance. My heart continually aches for him because I had to sit and watch as everything in his life was taken away, as he lost one friend after another, the death of his father, his grandfather and then watch as the second most important woman in his life, my sister and his favorite aunt in the world be taken by drugs, his grandfather by cancer and his dad from alcohol poisoning. His aunt died from complication of bacterial meningitis which she contracted from snorting pills that eventually caused a bacterial infection that went to her brain. She fought to live for thirteen months paralyzed from the neck down and then just as quickly as we thought she was beginning to get better she died just a few days after Christmas a year ago. My son has lost suffered greatly since early childhood, losing his best friend at fifteen, his dad at fourteen, his papaw at eighteen and his aunt at 28 and all to a deaths caused either by drugs or cancer causing chemicals such as tobacco. I can only pray that he will find that peace he so desperately needs in the Lord above so that he can conquer this disease and I know through prayer and faith it will all happen when the time is right and the Lord is ready to lift this affliction but I also realize that my son must want it and that he must also pray for it and I feel in my heart that he does. My son was arrested a few months ago, violation of probation for not attending probation and paying restitution. After beginning the Methadone treatment again he began to fall right back into his old ways and it wasn't long until he and the people he was with were getting pulled over by the police and within six months he found himself in jail. Now he is beginning to sober back up from the addiction he had fallen victim to once again and he is staring to see life as it truly is, nothing if we do not seek God in our darkest hour of need. When he was using again he would not listen to anyone who tried to lead him to Christ in order to help him but just as we all do during our journey down that dark and lonely path he thought he could do it alone and he found out that it just doesn't work that way. He is now sober and attending church and weekly bible study and he is *sending me scripture that the Lord has directed him to read in order to help him to see why these things happen and how we learn from our mistakes and that through our sufferings we become stronger when we do it for his Glory. My son now knows it was Christ who has brought him through this journey and that even though he was imprisoned it was all for a purpose much greater than he could see until now. It was the only way that God could show him that he could overcome the obstacles and that he was stronger than he ever believed for he had the Lord with him through it all, he only had to seek him and soak in the Word and his faith and the Lord raised him up from his affliction once again, He has never forsaken or abandoned us, His love is Merciful and Everlasting and he is with us always.*

What was the reason for my life ending up as a drug addict I really don't have the answer but I do have the answer to one thing and that is through my own addiction I pray that with the grace of God's help a leadership by using me as his vessel I may be able to help save other's from ever having to suffer the agonizing affliction in which I carried within my very soul for almost thirty years. My daughter tells me, Mom don't brag on me please, I'm not worthy of it, but what that baby girl of mine doesn't know she is now spreading the word of God through the direction in the path he has chosen He is the Light and the Way, He is the Life, Together let us choose to live through Christ Our Lord. Amen…

In all my travels through this long and sometimes lonely life I finally figured out that there has never been a moment that I was alone, the Lord and all his splendor has always been there beside me every step of the way, protecting me so that even when it seemed as though me or those I loved so deeply would be devoured by the hands of evil that constantly lurks within our shadows, he was always there to cast them back into the depths of darkness from where they had surfaced from in the beginning.

Evil Is Always Lurking

I began to remember that this wasn't the first time that the realms of evil had tried so violently to take over my earthly body to benefit its own desires. There had been a constant conspiracy from the dark forces that lie in waiting even from my earliest days of child hood. My sister Star and I were raised up in Tennessee at the foothills of the Great Smoky Mountains. We could walk outside on many occasions when we were visiting relatives or even our own homes as we got older and be faced with the most magnificent view in the world. The mountains in the summer were so green and so beautiful, you could sit in the evenings and watch the sunset and it was the most breath taking view ever and in the winter time the mountain tops would be snow covered peaks that looked like ice cream. The beauty of the mountains and the lakes was breath taking and we spent many summers camping and swimming in the nearby lakes while daddy would fish for hours sometimes catching nothing at all. Mom would lay and read, but I never knew how when her eyes were always fixated on us girls to keep us from drifting out to far so we didn't drown. We never learned to swim good enough to save ourselves because we were never allowed to go out past our waste and even though I took swim lessons at the local girls club I was so afraid by then I couldn't learn really for fear of drowning and of course she past this fear down to us so we were the same with our children, my daughter also took swim lessons but I couldn't watch so her dad taught her to swim and my son can swim some but not enough to save himself if he were drowning. Our Mother was one of those who always thought she could protect us from everything not ever even till this day facing that God is the only one who can truly protect from all things bad and that sometimes bad things must happen in order for good things to come of them. My experiences began at the early age of nine. The first time I ever saw anything was one night as I was going to get my Mom from her bedroom, I looked up and saw two women standing at the woodstove in the living room. I ran to Mom and woke her only for her to tell me it was just a shadow and to go back to sleep, but for years evil forces continued to come after me. I would go to bed and all the sudden a dark heavy shadow would rise up over my bed, terrified I would pray and cover my head and eventually fall asleep only to have it come after me. This force would hold me down on the bed with a force so strong that I was unable no matter how hard I tried to move to run to my mom or call out to her I couldn't and then when I did she would come running to the bedroom and it would be gone. This *happened to me until I grew up and left home and I knew then it was Satan trying to get me at my weakest point. After moving away from home it began to happen again a few years later only this time I saw him in the corner of the room and he told me he would be coming for me again. I moved from that place shortly thereafter. It seemed everyway he had tried to break me he had failed until the drugs came into my life. He was finally able to control me through the addiction but he also went after my younger sister too. We both had started out experimenting with alcohol but when the prescription opiates came into our lives they consumed us within a year. Star had always been the energetic one and I the laid back and rather lazy due to a childhood kidney disease and anemia so the opiates were my favorite because they gave me energy. Star like them all and would mix uppers with downers and eat far too many at a time which over the years caused her to accidentally overdose over a dozen times. There was no drug that she wouldn't try and I on the other hand would take nothing until I researched it and the effects of consuming the drug. I did not want to be an addict and tried so many times to stop throughout the years and did so many times only to fall right back into the cycle but my sister was just the opposite, even though I know deep down she would have loved to have been able to stop, she just couldn't. I went back home after moving away to South Carolina a few times after talking her into checking herself into rehab only to have our Mom to go and check her right back out thinking that she could save her when in all reality she was no more than her co-dependent.*

Eventually my addiction got so severe that I truly realized I had to stop but by that time I was so physically sick with Arthritis and Fibromyalgia that I had to have pain killers to function and have any quality of life or be able to work. I decided then that I would begin treatment at the local Methadone clinic for I knew that if I continued to take the opiates I would die. I began the treatment in 2008 and after a year I was back out in the work force that I had not been able to return to for over seven years due to my addiction. I suggested it to my Mother for my sister but she refused to listen and a short while later, I discovered my sister had Hepatitis C and would be starting Inferon treatments for the disease. All of her years of addiction had caused her liver to disease and now she would be fighting to live and beat the disease before it turned to cirrhosis of the liver. For over a year she went through the treatments but to everyone's disappointment it didn't work. It finally got to the point that Star got so bad on the pills that she would get cut out from every doctor she went to for her condition because she was so addicted and so immune to the pills and low milligrams that they would write her prescriptions and she would eat them all up in just a few short days and begin harassing the doctors for more so they would discontinue treating her. This went on for many years to the point that she started to make up disease she had and find a new doctor and lie saying that at one time she had Multiple Sclerosis so she could get highly potent pain killers. They did brain scans and saw lesions on the brain but what they didn't know those had been there for years from her being beaten by ex-husbands and jumping out of moving vehicles just to go to the E.R. for drugs. I tried desperately to tell my Mother the truth but she refused to accept it and that was when she truly became my sister's co-dependent. During this time my Mother also was becoming addicted to pain killers and nerve pills. She had let her baby sister convince her that she had Fibromyalgia and went to a quack specialist who push around on her pressure points and diagnosed her with the disease. When I would try to tell her she too was becoming an addict she would defend herself by saying the doctor gives them to me for this terrible pain but she had never complained of the pain before and she worked standing on concrete floors every day and had been in several car accidents which would have explained some of her pain but it seemed when she and my stepfather split was when she decided she was sick. A year or so later my Mom finally realized she too was addicted but just like my sister refused to stop or even try to stop taking the pills.

The day after Thanksgiving 2010 I would have to say was one of the worst days of my life. I was looking on my face book account when I saw a cousin's status that said my sister was in A Tennessee Trauma unit and they didn't think she would make it through the night. I hadn't spoken to them in a couple of months because it had gotten to the point that my sister never answered her phone because my niece said she was always high and passed out and my anger at Mother because she wouldn't try to get her into rehab had gotten me to the point I dreaded calling because Mom would always try to make me feel guilty by telling me I needed to come home and take care of Star. I had tried but Mothers interference wouldn't let me. I face booked my cousin to see where my sister was and to find out what was wrong that was when I was informed she had some kind of infection on the brain and was unresponsive. I immediately phone The University of Tennessee Medical Center Surgical Care unit and spoke to my step father who broke into tears and kept telling me he was so sorry. What do you mean what did you do I ask? Apparently my sister had been very ill for over a month and a half to the point she had to be carried and screamed with headaches continuously. That morning she had collapsed on the kitchen floor at Mothers house and had become paralyzed and unable to speak. She was rushed to the local E.R. where she was air lifted to the trauma center where she had been taken directly into emergency surgery and was then diagnosed with Bacterial Meningitis. She was in a coma and a shunt was placed in her brain to try to pull the fluid which the nuero surgeon had said lay almost an inch think on her brain and CDEC was called in out of Atlanta. They did not expect her to make it through the night. That night I picked my daughter up and we headed out for Tennessee praying my sister would be ok. We arrived at the hospital around 4 the next morning after driving all night and I walked over and touched my Mother who was sleeping in the waiting area. I was not nor do I think I could have ever been prepared for what I was faced with next. There in room number eight lay the body of someone almost unrecognizable. My sister was on life support and part of her hair had been shaved away for the surgery in which they had placed the stint on her brain. Her face was swollen to that of a basketball and her brain had so much fluid on it that it was leaking from her eyes and ears. I was so angry as my Mother began to speak because my sister had been ill for weeks and weeks and they should have had her here long before now. I was even told my Mother had tried to get the medics to carry my sister back to bed instead of taking her to the hospital because my family had thought she was just pill sick because she had went to two local hospitals and because of her reputation as a drug addict they had sent her home. One doctor had even went as far to tell her she had antibiotics at home and she could treat herself just as well at home as they could in the hospital. If they had even have bothered to do a spinal tap at either one of the times my sister was admitted to these two hospitals she would more than likely still be with us today. Although addiction is a very common disease among people in Tennessee,, it doesn't mean that local physicians have the right to turn their backs on anyone whether it be an addict or the President of the United States. Yes, my sister was neglected by the medical professionals in both local hospitals in which she was treated because of her passed history but I believe these people should be held accountable for neglecting to do the proper procedures that are called for when a patient is admitted with even the slightest possibility that the illness could be Meningitis. My sister had lost 20 lbs. during her two month illness, she complained of a constant headache and sensitivity to light and she even had two major seizures, the last while walking through the grocery store. The physicians were told of these and still did nothing to test her even when they were told she was too weak to walk from my Mother's house to the car and had to be carried by her son. All of the symptoms were there yet not one medical expert took the time to do a twenty minute procedure that would have determined life or death for Star. The more I heard from everyone as to the events leading up to this very moment the more furious I became. For two months my sister had tried to tell everyone that something was terribly wrong but nobody would listen except for her daughter Jessie and furious. As I walked out of the unit I was face to face with my sister's pride and joy, her little girl, my sweet niece Jessie who was thirteen years old and terrified. Jess the one who had begged my Mother to take my sister to Knoxville because she knew just how ill Star truly was, the one who even though she was still just a child had been forced to sit time after time and babysit Star when she was so wasted away on pills that Jessie thought she would die. At that moment I was so stricken with guilt that it was all I could do to look this precious child in the face but I knew I had to be strong for her now more than ever. If only I hadn't left them and moved so far away, if I had taken them with me and gotten Star into a treatment facility away from our Mother, if I had called more often or went home to visit more. All of the if's could do nothing for her now and if I hadn't moved away when I did I would have probably been dead by this time due to my own addiction that had plummeted out of control when I learned of my Dad's terminal lung cancer. My heart was telling me that what I did, I did to protect my life and for the love of my family, but what about Star and Jessie. They were my family too and now we were being faced with the possibility that Star would not survive this Silent Killer because according to the CDC" Center for Disease Control" in Atlanta Star the infection had been building up for over a period of possibly two months and if it had not been for the intravenous antibiotics she had received at the previous hospitals she would have died much sooner ;however because they were not the right drugs for the infection that lay in a large puddle on her brain the once curable infection had turned lethal leaving Star paralyzed completely from the neck down and unable to breathe on her own and all of this was due to her reputation as a drug addict because of the doctors who had over the past two months before releasing her from the hospitals would still prescribe her very powerful painkillers which was something each and every one of them had been doing for over the past 17 years. When she learned to work and manipulate the system and the doctors she was able to get the most powerful pain killers on the market today such as Opana, Roxycodone, Morphine, and then she was also prescribed Medications for conditions that she didn't even have and due to the negligence of the prescribing physicians there were no test done to prove any existed. She made up a story, researched or met people who had multiple sclerosis, lupus, fibromyalgia, rheumatoid arthritis, high blood pressure and she would find a doctor who was popular for writing out prescriptions for those drugs and she would go in for her appointment looking like she was on the brink of death. I thought that when Daddy began to get worse with his cancer that it would help me and her to get sober but it did just the opposite, we began to medicate to numb the pain. My back hurt so badly from lifting and tugging on Daddy and I tried to keep my home disinfected all the time because I had heard that people who live with those who have terminal lung cancer and pulmonary disease get infections themselves. We were a family on a dead end street not knowing who would be next in line to become the victim of this also famous family killer due to either being a smoker or by being subjected to second hand smoke on a daily basis. It became so very clear on that day that the one thing my family had not been doing was, Living in the Word, the word of God. Giving our lives to him completely and allowing him to provide and care for all that was ailing us. Though we had good doctors providing round the clock care for my sister, she was a patient in a research/student medical facility where people learn to become doctors and surgeons. The hospital had never been known for having a good reputation for saving lives and the whole time my sister was in Surgical Critical Care 1 in every three were taken off of life support and most because the doctors told the family they would never recover. I wonder how many of those people would be walking around today had they been given the chance to heal and have been treated like a patient instead of just a bed waiting to become available. How many of these beautiful precious lives would be here today had the family and the doctors had enough faith if only that the size of a mustard seed to be filled with the hope and faith that the Gracious, Loving God whom we prayed to daily for that miracle healing would have answered those prayers if we had only been a little more patient and have never let the dark forces of evil creep into our minds to instill that one little moment of doubt and encircled us with those working for the evil one so that in a moment of only a piece of the question what if or maybe they want get well stole from you all the faith and hope and belief that all things were possible with our Heavenly Father in control. I by no means am saying that every person who lay in that unit would have come out of the coma and lived life as if nothing had ever happened but I am saying that in those days and months that followed as my sister lay there and fought to live with every ounce of strength God had given her we did not truly begin to see the unbelievable change until she was transferred to a small Christian Community Hospital that sat back in the country surrounded by the most beautiful splendor and peaceful tranquility That filled your lungs with the cleanest, purest air I had breathed in quiet awhile. The hospital was our last hope because all others had been convinced by the University Of Tennessee Medical Center that Star was in a vegetative state and that there was no possible chance for recovery. When Star entered Jellico Community Hospital she weighed a small, frail and ghastly looking 62 lbs. The face that once held the beauty of a prima donna was now nothing but pale sunken cheek bones and her hair was falling out due to the malnutrition in which she was suffering at that point. Star was taken directly to Intensive Care where she was met by a staff of Christian nurses who fell in love with her instantly. There was Kathy, Latisha, and others and then Dr. Tin. Who worked fiercely to get Star in stable condition and work to get her gaining weight and within two months she had gained up to just over a hundred pounds and she had begun to drink out of a straw and was eating solid foods. One morning as my Mother and my niece were standing across the room they heard a faint, yet strong voice say "I want a cup of coffee." Looking at each other in disbelief they turned to my sister and once again Star said a little louder I want a cup of coffee. I could just imagine the two of them trying to climb over each other to get to the nurse to tell her what Star had said, and sure enough she got her very first cup of coffee in almost seven months. Star was getting stronger and stronger by the day and on good days she was able to breathe on her own for hours at a time. The doctor was convinced that she would be weaned from the respirator within the year. In October my daughter came in from Alabama for a short break in the fall and we made a surprise visit to Tennessee. Mom said that was the greatest day ever as she watched me walked into the I.C.U where my sister lay, she looked up to see me and my daughter and her face lit up as bright as the Northern Star the night baby Jesus entered this world. The light that radiated around her gave a glow so bright that her eyes seemed as blue as the brightest sapphire and the smile that lit up her face was one of such excitement and love that I honestly thought my heart would truly explode. The happiness that filled that hospital unit that day was not just that of my family but of every nurse and caregiver within the unit. We laughed and Star tried over and over to tell the nurse that her sister wanted to stay the night but the nurse kept thinking she was saying scissors and that was when I decided to break the ice with my cute little joke from our childhood saying so you want some scissors so sledge can cut your hair again lie when I cut it off to the scalp when you were little to try and get rid of your cowlick. Everyone exploded into laughter including Star, she laughed until she literally wore herself out and we had scared Mom to death because she was afraid all the laughter would hurt her. Oh dear Mother I tried to explain, this is just what she needed, HAPPINESS, LAUGHTER, JOY, and the presence of God's Love all up in that room that day. It wasn't long after the two hours of non- stop hysteria that Star went to sleep from utter exhaustion. I was able to wake her briefly before leaving that afternoon but I can say today without any hesitation, I saw the Love of God all around Star's room that day. She was happy and she was in such a peaceful place that I almost felt I could pick her up and carry her out and everything would be absolutely fine. The light that radiated from her that day gave me the comfort that I need to know that she was exactly where she needed to be at this moment in time. There was a miracle in the making that day and all I could do was pray that everyone else had seen the wonder that shone all around us that day. I prayed and tried so very hard to get everyone to just let any doubt or any hesitation go from their minds and to let the Lord Almighty fill them up with his presence, to believe with all their hearts and all their souls that soon Star would surprise everyone when she recovered despite what the other hospital and all its specialist had said, for they had *not witnessed what we had all seen today and from that day forward Star's condition began to improve remarkably. She was eating solid foods such as gravy and biscuits for breakfast, chicken nuggets, milkshakes, all the foods she loved she was eating her fair share and with that came her strength. There was still a long way to go but with God it was going to be alright and I truly believed this with all my heart and soul.*

Around the second week of November Star began to show signs of swelling on the brain once again. This wasn't the first time this had happened but the problem with it happening at this facility was that there wasn't a neuro surgeon that could care for her condition. The Dr. began making phone calls to try to get her transferred to a facility equipped to care for the hydracephilitis that was causing the flood to gather on Star brain. Her heart rate was elevated and her temperature was beginning to elevate up to 101-102-103 and they had to pack her in the cooling blanket. I was on the phone and talking to a neurosurgeon at Mercy Hospital in Columbia South Carolina who agreed to take my sister and I phone my Mother immediately to let her know the wonderful news, but she had gotten the hospital to get the insurance to agree to transport Star to Oakridge Medical another hospital that was not equipped to treat this type of Traumatic Brain Injury. Upon transporting Star to Oakridge her hospital documentation was mixed up and she was admitted as vegetative just as she was the day she was exited from The University of Tennessee Medical and guess that the hospital was that was relaying the information to the Oakridge

Nero Specialist, none other than University of Tennessee. When Jellico Community found out that the paperwork had been mixed up they immediately came to Star's rescue; however, because of the hydracephalitis and the amount of fluid that was rapidly gathering on her Brain, Star was beginning to drift in and out of consciousness. Dr. Tinn was on the phone with the hospital constantly and the nurses made it a point to come to the hospital to try to get these specialists to see that Star was making remarkable progress in her recovery but they refused to listen. My niece and I even showed them home movies we had made at the hospital in Jellico just days before she became ill and the Dr. whom I believe to have been from the U.K. according to her accent looked at them and shrugged her shoulders stating that a three year old could do those things. I ask her if a three year old would remember her son and daughter and where she lived and first and foremost her Sister Sledge, the nickname she had given me at the age of somewhere around her late thirties. Her reply was we will wait and see what happens. It was Dec.27th and I ask Star if she was going to be alright, she shrugged her shoulders and gave me a kiss and I promised her it would be ok. I had to leave that night to return to South Carolina and back to work and I honestly thought that this hospital would see they had made a mistake and put the shunt back into Stars brain and draw the fluid off, but I had never been more wrong. On December 29th my niece phone me hysterical begging me to get back as soon as possible or they were going to turn my sisters life support off. My Mom got the phone and tried to convince me that *my sister was gone that there was nothing there but I tried to tell her the same thing had happened at U.T when she first became ill and they said she had a severe stroke that had damaged the whole left side of her brain, it was then that they began to do everything but hold a gun on my family to make them cut life support. I begged Mom not to do anything until I could get there, but just thirty minutes after I hung up the phone my sister was taken off of life support and left this world. Star was gone too soon because the people who said they loved her the most lacked the one thing they needed the most and that was "FAITH" faith that all things are possible with God. I also realized too, that as we prayed for her recovery and for her to get well and to be able to go home that even though it did not happen as we all had hoped for it too. Star did get to go home, she went home to the Lord, I honestly believe he knew if he let her go back to the life she had known before the illness, she would have ended right back in the relentless, unforgiving, cycle with the battle of the addiction that had placed her in the situation that had taken her life as she had known it before. In that moment of my own selfishness I realized God had saved her, she was now free from pain, free from the constant battle and agonizing torture she had endured for so many years, the endless nights she had lay in bed begging God to just ease the pain, to take it all away. I realized that day even through my anger towards my Mom for not seeing the signs, to my step father for not making her go to a good hospital and then I remembered all the times before when she had cried wolf and we would all jump in the car to* get her to the hospital thinking she was dying or something was terribly wrong, only to find out she was in need of a fix because she was dope sick. I realized that Jellico Community Hospital was Star's saving grace, it was the place she went to make her peace with God and to fully accept him as her Lord and Savior. If I ever believe anything it will be that my sister found God inside the room of that Intensive Care Unit surrounded by her earthly angels who kept watch over her both day and night until God made his final decision to truly save her life and to give her everlasting life that she could spend eternity with him in Heaven and with this my heart rejoiced and I now find myself waiting anxiously for the day when we can all be reunited once again so I can take off running from one side and she by the other and we will meet in the middle hugging and kissing one another and rejoicing in the presence of our Father God. You see, I realized that day when God took her home, sometimes even though it hurts us unimaginably God takes us to prevent something much worst from happening to us later down the road. I hope Star is watching down over me now and seeing that I am thinking of her all the time and praying that her story, our story, hers, mine, the whole family will in some way help those who are struggling the battle of prescription addiction, molestation, abuse, and all forces of darkness in the journey of the Serpents Sting that they may rise up and raise their hands to the heavens to the Lord Almighty that we can conquer all evil temptations no matter how tempting it seems, how sweet it smells or how pleasant it promises to make you feel. REMEMBER EVIL TEMPTATION LIES, It KNOWS NO

TRUTH AND ONCE IT HAS YOU WRAPPED WITHINH IT"S GRASP YOU WILL SUFFER A TORMENT GREATER THAN YOU COULD EVER POSSIBLY BEGIN TO IMAGINE.. Please my brothers and sisters today ask yourself, do you want to live life with the evil darkness that is waiting for you to give your life to Satan to suffer eternal damnation in the lake of fire or to call out to the Lord, to accept Jesus Christ as your one and only Savior, to know that he died on the cross for you and me so that we can have everlasting life with him in the Kingdom of Heaven. Accept him today for he is the Way, the Truth and the Light of all Salvation.

And Then There Was Mother

After I was grown and had left home to begin my own life it wasn't long until my mom and dad divorced. My Dad was devastated and for the years that followed I watched as he grieved himself into a world of deep depression and the longing to have the woman he loved to just take him back, to give him another chance, but as bad as I hurt for my parents, their divorce was the best thing for my mom for she hadn't been happy for many years. Mom had made a promise that as long as I was at home she would not leave dad and she kept her word. Within that first year after I moved out she filed for a divorce and began to make a new life for herself. She began working and bought a car and learned to drive. She was determined to make it on her own as a single Mother and she did just that. She worked and provided for my younger sister and still continued to care for my Grandmother whose health deteriorated more with each passing year. Mom had begun a relationship with her first teenage crush and she was on top of the world, she was free and didn't have to answer to anyone for the first time in over 21 years. She began to live like a 38 year old woman instead of an old home body who cooked, cleaned and took care of everyone except herself. I was so glad to finally see her truly happy. In the summer of 1985 the man whom my Mother had been dating ever since her divorce was in a terrible automobile accident that left him clinging to life. Mother was devastated. As the days turned into weeks and the weeks into months he lay in a coma hooked up to life support. One evening his trach had slipped away from the opening in his throat and he went without oxygen to his brain for over five minutes due to either neglect by the attending nurses not checking when his alarm sounded or because the alarm had malfunctioned and not gone off at all. He was pronounced brain dead and the family unhooked him from life support but he didn't die instead he continued to breathe on his on for many months until he finally died of other complications due to the trauma which had occurred from the accident. His best friend had been there for my mom during that whole year and a half and with that they began to grow close which eventually stirred up a romance that would prove to be both beautiful and horrible. They are still together today after many ups and downs. Being wealthy and losing everything but each other and then beginning to build it all back up again. I always looked at my Mother as one of the strongest women I had ever known. She despised medicine with a *passion, especially pain killers because she had watched them turn my Grandmother into an addict and it was just too much for her to have to deal with at time, especially when my Grandma would phone pleading death at two in the morning and my Mother would rush to her side only to realize she was out of her pain medication and needed a pill to ease her withdraw symptoms. I never saw my Mother take anything stronger than an aspirin all of my life until the year 1999 when the doctor told her she had Fibromyalgia and began prescribing her Hydrocodone and Xanax along with muscle relaxers and sleeping pills and it just continued down the same path me, my sister, our Grandmother, aunts and now my mom had fallen victim to the Serpents Sting too. She didn't truly understand all of the stories I had confided in her about my own addiction as well as my sisters until the day came when she ran out of her pain medication a couple of weeks early. She ended up in bed fighting the fight we had fought ourselves for so many years. Just as I had sworn to never take another pain pill as long as I lived I listened as my Mother repeated those exact words to me, yet as soon as it came time to get another prescription she was there at the pharmacy anxiously awaiting to get her hands on the bottles just as we had done before her and yet she still continued to make excuses for her addiction saying but I am sick and I hurt. Well mom so were we and that is why 20 years later I was still fighting to not only get sober which I had done several times but to stay sober and I had realized long ago that is easier said than done. It has now been fourteen years since my Mother first began using opiates for pain and* she wonders why they don't wor anymore, She runs out early every month and it is my stepfather who gives her most of his medication so she won't go into cardiac arrest due to her blood pressure rising so high from no medication. I don't know the woman I use to call my Mother anymore, she is a complete stranger who lays in bed most of the day and roams the house at night. She gets so wasted on the medication that her speech gets slurred and she too nods out. It breaks my heart to see the woman who once had the spirit of a wild stallion digging through drawers looking for a nerve pill she may have dropped or a pain pill she may have over looked. I get so angry because the woman who ridiculed me and told me she couldn't believe she had raised a daughter who was weak when I first confronted her of my addiction at 23 is now the exact replica of the young woman who came to her for support all those years ago I now want to say to her, I can't believe I have a Mother who finally after fifty years fell into the devils trap when she new better. I listen to her still to this day put others down for their misfortunes and acting like she has done nothing wrong. I wonder sometimes did she unknowingly suffer a break down that we didn't notice because she was always so stern, ill and loved misery that she honestly doesn't realize the mistakes she has made. I wish I could answer that with a yes but it would be a lie for she remembers too many things from her childhood and previous years to be crazy. My Mother has always been a control freak, if she couldn't have some kind of control over you then she chose not to come around much at all and I am not one to be *controlled so this has caused my children and I a significant amount of pain and hurt because it was so easy for her to act like we didn't exist at all until my sister died. I pray that Mother finds peace in this life for she is one of the most miserable women I have ever known but she is getting older and it just seems with each year that passes she continues to find something knew to help continue to wallow in misery. I was lucky to have had both parents growing up and I loved both of them equally but it is hard when you feel there is nothing you could ever do that would make your Mother proud. I never once remember her telling me that she was proud of me or that I had done a good job as a Mother, daughter, sister or anything else but I have forgiven it all as I have grown older though I will never forget the hurt I will always love my Mother and I wish she could stop the medications just to see how sick they are actually making her but I feel it is too late to try for fear it could kill her. I pray God keeps her close in his loving grace and eases her burdened heart so that her remaining days may be pleasant and filled with love for Christ and all of us who love and miss the woman she once was. I remember telling her before she ever took the first pill that addiction knows no prejudice, it will take anyone and any age and destroy them. I think she now understands what I was trying to tell her all those years ago. I remember when my sister and I use to say to one another how we wished she could feel what we felt just once when we were drug sick and she would curse and yell or tell us how week or how pathetic we were, well that was one wish I truly wish had not came true. I didn't* honestly mean it nor did Star. We were two dope sick daughters of a woman who had watched her own Mother suffer from addiction for the most part of her life so why wouldn't she be angry when the two children she had birthed had fallen into the same cycle. We didn't realize just how much our Mother had suffered both emotionally and physically or how much her heart had been broken as she watched the woman she loved with all of her heart being slowly eaten alive by prescription pain killers, valium and as she got older and weaker due to several open heart surgeries that left her heart lying within her chest cavity like a raw piece of hamburger meat because the cardiologist had to remove the protective pouch from around her heart when he performed as he said, "The Last heart surgery that he could ever do to her because there were no more procedures that could be done," three thyroid surgeries, a radical mastectomy on her right breast under local anesthetic, because the physician said she would not wake up if she was put under for an extended amount of time, so they basically chopped her breast off as quickly as they possibly could, biopsied and stitched her back together in an attempt to save her life after finding she had breast cancer during a routine mammography. My Grandmother was a very proud woman and by that I mean she went to great efforts when she was well to look the best she could. She would bathe and use talcum powders and lotions and I will always remember her lovely scent, she always smelled of jasmine. She would open her closet and there she kept scented sachet pouches that she hung on hangers plus she would spray her Jasmine *perfume to in order to ensure her clothes always smelled so good. I use to laugh hysterically at her because she kept her panties and bras in a suitcase under her bed and she would get me to get it out so she could open it and spray her under garments with her jasmine perfume. I ask her one time why she kept them in that blue suitcase that was pushed pretty far up under her bed and she replied, "I want to make sure the moths don't eat them up." I remember thinking sure Mamaw,* knew it was because deep in the back of her mind she was afraid someone was going to steal those silk granny panties if she put them in the drawers where they belonged. God love her, my Grandmother suffered from severe emotional problems that probably stemmed from the nervous breakdown she suffered after the birth of her twelfth child, a beautiful premature little blonde haired, blue eyed baby girl who weighed a little over three pounds in February of 1952. In those days it was a miracle if children survived when born that premature and that small. Just about all women breast fed but due to the early arrival of Brenda Joyce Williams there were no little bottles or little bottle nipples and my Grandmother had no milk plus one of her nipples was introverted. Brenda was kept in the hospital due to her size and fed with a dropper and then when she went home my Grandmother made sugar tits for her to suck. I don't really know exactly when the breakdown occurred but honestly I don't know how Mamaw had kept from having more than one after having that many children and all of them at home except for two and that meant she had them naturally with no anesthetic. To me my Grandmother was a, "Hell of a woman." Even after having twelve children, being basically poverty stricken, living in what people refer to even today as the Spoons' old two story haunted house I suppose because they could get it for cheaper rent and it was a very large brick home. Haunted or not it was big enough for a family of fourteen.. I have listened to the stories from my aunts and uncle over the years as they would tell stories about the unexplainable events that took place when they lived in that house and I would have ran away from home before I would have lived in that old house which for no apparent reason burned to the ground several years ago. What was really weird was the fact that hot spots kept popping up for over a week after the fire and the fire department would have to go back out to the site and wet it down to keep the fire from blazing back out of control which could have caused the neighboring homes to catch fire. It was really strange because there were no winds that would have caused that to happen and the entire home had literally burned to the ground and the only thing that was left standing was the chimney and that was where the hot spots would generate from every time 911 was called. The Fire Marshall said he had never seen anything like it. Could my Grandmother perhaps have been taken emotional hostage by the evil forces that had terrorized everyone living in that old house? My Grandfather built their home when his Father gave him a piece of land that would be just over the hill from my Great Grandparents. It was a little white house with two bedrooms. It may have been little but it was theirs. The older boys and girls married and left home to start families of their own. There were now four children until my Grandmother had the last two which were both premature and lucky to have survived. I can understand how my Grandmother lost her mind. Her last child was conceived just as she had begun to go through menopause and that was when my Mother had been forced to quit school at the age of eleven. This has also helped me to better understand some of my own mom's emotional instabilities as I have gotten older. My heart actually began to ache for her in knowing that her childhood was cut short due to my Grandmothers breakdown and extremely poor health. Mom was left to play the role of Mother to her four younger siblings and in fifty one years I have never heard her once say she regretted having to quit school or that she hated having to raise her younger siblings instead of being able to play like most eleven years old girls do. She told me stories of how her fourth grade school teacher had tried to force her to write right handed because mom was what they called a south paw, she was left handed. I can only imagine how my mom had felt being told you weren't normal if you weren't right handed back in those days. I was later cursed with the same teacher my mom had when I too went into the fourth grade. When I told her who I was and that Virginia Williams was my Mother I remember her saying oh she is. I could tell then it was going to be a long year but I didn't realize just how long it was actually going to be because that was the year I was diagnosed with the kidney disease My handwriting had always been very pretty and very neat. I had always gotten A's for my writing in my other classes from kindergarten thru third grade until Mrs. Roberts. My first grade card she gave me a C in handwriting. When my Mother saw that grade she went ballistic. She picked the phone up and made the call, I do not remember what was said that day as my Mother spoke to her twenty years later woman to woman and that is probably for the best but I was treated very differently and never made anything other than A's in handwriting. That day my Mother had turned the table on that mean old woman and mom became the intimidator and was treated with the upmost respect from my teacher from that day forward and when I became very ill with the kidney disease shortly thereafter Ms. Roberts phoned to check on me often, she had the class make get well cards and when I was finally allowed to return to school in mid Spring after being on homebound teaching Ms. Roberts watched over me like she was my Grandmother. I wished my Grandmother could have gotten around like this woman. Between her sickness and her depression she stayed hidden away in her bedroom where it was so dark you couldn't see your hand in front of your face. I spent many nights with her when I became a teenager so that my mom could stay home and be a mom to my sister and my Grandmother loved for me to stay. She would lock us in her bedroom and we would talk about all of her kids and their children and when we ran out of stuff to talk about we would make stuff up. She kept a 20 gauge shotgun sitting beside her bed loaded and ready to shoot if she had to and she was a pro at it she could hit anything and would not hesitate to do so if the situation ever arose. During those years I didn't realize just how paranoid she truly was. She would wake me up out of a dead sleep and say" did you hear them Tisha they are out there again". I would sit up and listen hoping she wouldn't hear my teeth chattering from fear, but I never heard anyone. I now wonder if she didn't just do those things because she couldn't sleep and didn't want to sit there alone in the dark because when I looked back on it she had done my mom the same way even going as far to call her in the middle of the night and tell her she was sick just so mom would go out. It was such a sad life that Mamaw lived and I truly wish I had known then just had bad everything truly was and maybe I could have helped more, done more, maybe it would have been what saved me from my own addiction and failures in my life; however, it didn't happen that way so I must take it from here, today, and live the rest of my life fighting to stay afloat and out of the grasp of the evil that once held on so tightly that I never thought escape was possible and even though I must still take medication today for pain and emotional disorders and a lot due to the side effects of so many years of my drug addiction. The arthritis is so bad I cannot sleep in bed anymore because I go stiff and have to have someone get me up because my lower back goes so stiff I cannot bend into a sitting position to get up so I sleep in a recliner. The sad part of beginning to recover from years of addiction is thinking you are going to be as good as new, never realizing that you have grown older, weaker and that you will never feel like you remembered before your addiction began. The great news is you can start to correct so many of the wrongs. A good daily regimen of nutrition and exercise will strengthen your body and you will begin to feel youthful again and realize that the natural high is much greater and so much more enjoyable than the addiction could have ever been. I suffer from chronic fatigue syndrome and there are literally days when it is all I feel I can do to get up and walk to the bathroom but then I say to myself, "you can do it" and you can, you are more capable than you give yourself credit, {for example}.. remember when you were an addict and so drug sick you couldn't get out of bed, how you kicked and thrashed around as if you were going to die at any moment, and then when you found out where to get a fix you flew out of bed like you had sprouted wings and ran to the car and drove off like an Indy racecar driver to get that fix. It is all up to you my friend! You have the will power and are capable of so much when it is something you truly want and when sobriety becomes that important to you this is the time you will succeed and when the Lord is allowed and invited into your life he will hold you and comfort you and make that journey more bearable than trying to do it alone, for when you try to do it without him most of the time you will not succeed because you have nothing to keep you grounded. God's Love is real, it is true, His Love is stronger than any addiction, or any obstacle that will ever be thrown in your path. When you allow him to take charge of your thoughts, your feelings, your heart and your soul, then you will see how beautiful life truly is. Each day that passes as I continue my road to recovery, I become closer and closer to my Lord, he gives me the strength and the courage I need to make the right decisions and to stay on the right path. I know now that I will make it and I will conquer this disease that has tried so desperately to destroy my entire family for over three generations because I don't know how many of my ancestors were afflicted before I ever knew what was really happening. I know now that I will survive and with God by my side this next year will be the year that I will be able to hold my head high and look toward the morning when I can shout out, I WON!!!!

Aunt Brenda Please Don't Die

Brenda Joyce Williams Fletcher, the youngest of twelve and my Mother's baby sister. After dropping out of high school her junior year to go out into the working world and to marry her great love Kenneth, she had two beautiful daughters and lived a cozy but simple life loving her husband and kids with all her heart. Brenda worked for a corporation that made pistons for motor vehicles and was exposed to a potent cleaning chemical that would eventually cause her to develop a severe lung disease that would prove to be almost fatal. She stood on concrete floors for eight to ten hours a day for over 20 years which caused the varicose vein in one leg to become so shattered and torn that the pain was almost unbearable. She ate prescription Ibprofen like candy until it no longer relieved the pain. Brenda was the first to be diagnosed with Fibromyalgia in1997 it seemed that anyone who had unexplainable pain where there was no evidence of ruptured disc, torn muscles or anything that could be detected on x-ray that you were beginning to be diagnosed with this somewhat new disease. The big problem was that when they diagnosed you with it the doctors instantly began prescribing massive quantities of very potent pain killers. Brenda began taking loratab but because she said they made her sick and wasn't strong enough she went straight to the devil, "oxycontin" For sixteen years I watched as this powerful, toxic pain killer slowly killed my aunt. Brenda had been a very large woman for over twenty years but around the age of 40 she lost over a hundred pounds and became a sexy little blonde with beautiful blue eyes and the whitest teeth and a personality you loved to be around. She was vivacious, loved to dance and party all night. After her divorce from her husband of over twenty years she went a little wild, fell in love with a local man and they were in a serious relationship for quite a few years then the next thing I knew she no longer that happy go lucky woman but someone who lay in bed wallowing in misery from the pain and burning of this disease called fibromyalgia. She continued taking these drugs for sixteen years but in early 2012 she almost died due to an almost accidental overdose of medication and the inability to breathe on her own. I knew it was going to happen eventually but that didn't make the pain any easier to bare. Brenda was only ten years older than me and what was so bad was that the doctors never once told her that all the medications that they were prescribing her would eventually kill her either by shutting down her respitory system or by causing liver disease, renal failure or all of these, so in 2012 she was placed on life support at the local hospital and the family was told they didn't know if she would survive. Brenda was placed in a drug induced coma for the life support and then she awoke and everyone was elated but she had to get over the oxycontin addiction. I remember listening to her breathe and it sounding like chains rattling in a scary movie and wanting to tell her it was the medication as well as the lung disease causing this but I knew if I did she would blame it all on her previous job and never admit it was the pain killers because that's what addicts do. We will blame every illness or accident on everything but the true culprit, 'Our Addiction." Brenda was transferred to a Nursing Home when she became somewhat strong enough to leave the hospital and she promised God that if he would let her live she would never take another oxycontin again and to this day she has been free of opiates for over six months now "Praise God." I saw her over Labor Day when I went back home for the holiday and she looked wonderful, she has gotten to be a very large woman again but it is mainly due to the large amounts of sterroids she has to take in order to be able to breathe. .I am so thankful that she is alive! because she could have easily died and not gotten to experience that freedom from the miserable evil that had taken control of her very being. That little pill had become her life link and without it she would suffer pain more brutal than any she had ever known. She now takes ibuprofen like before and a drug designed especially for nerve pain and fibromyalgia called lyrica and she is doing amazingly great. She whispered to me that people just don't know do they Tisha and I shook my head and replied no honey they don't and I hope that many of them never have to find out. Amen to that she replied. The day my precious Aunt Brenda stopped breathing, she took a journey into the light and saw our Lord and all his love that surrounded her and at that moment she realized just how precious life truly is and how fortunate we all are to be blessed with not only our life but all that goes with it, our two arms, two legs with which to stand, two feet with which to walk, to eyes with which we see and she realized how much we actually take it all for granted and on that day her life changed forever. Brenda decided to live her life for God, to live each day as if it were her last and to know that when this life is over there is a splendid, spectacular place that we can only begin to imagine its beauty in which will be our new home in our new bodies where we will live happily for all eternity. I saw that peace and His Light shining brightly within her that night and I knew then that she was going to be just fine for she had been truly filled with the Holy Spirit.

Cousins are not excluded

For anyone to ever think evil only attacks certain people they could not be more wrong and addiction knows no prejudice. Coming from such a large family it is hard to have imagined a childhood without anyone to play with. There were so many cousins that a Saturday at my Grandparents house looked like a family reunion. Some of us *visited more than others but it was mostly due to the fact that we lived so close to my Grandparents, either next door or just out the road within walking distance. I was particularly close to Ricky and Tony who were my Mother's oldest brother's children and Tony was a year my senior my senior and Ricky was about four years older. They were two mischievous boys. Tony shot himself in the leg before he was even a teenager because he had a gun stuck down his pants and Ricky ran to Grans to get my Mom. I remember how scared Ricky was that his little brother was going to die. They had been arguing over a glass of tea that day. Over the years they still just as brothers do bickered about something all the time. They both always thought they were right when probably neither was but that's what brothers and sisters do. Ricky began experimenting with drugs as a teenager. His Father had raised them in church up until they went to live with their Grandparents as teenagers. Pot and alcohol were the first drugs and then of course he met people while partying that led to acid and shroons as well as THC and later cocaine and then at eighteen he suffered a terrible motorcycle accident that totally crushed his leg and after hours of surgery and traction and a full body cast. Ricky became addicted to pain killers for the first time and this led to a lifetime of battling his addiction. From the age of 18 to his death in 2009 Ricky had fought to survive, we spoke of it often and how we wished we had never done any of it and how the doctors just prescribe all of these drugs to you knowing all to well that if administered for extended periods of time you will become addicted. I found a way out through so* much research and by my son choosing outpatient treatment that helped me to begin the road to recovery and I only wish my loved ones who have died due to the sting of the evil serpent had of known that there was a way to win the battle if that was what they truly wanted.

Something about Missy

I have encountered many people since first beginning my outpatient treatment but none of them have touched my heart as much as that of a young woman named Missy Like so many others she too suffers from addiction but her story is one that breaks my heart and makes me want to take today's society of parents and beat them into the world of reality, so many of today's kid's end up as addicts due to their parent's addiction. The parents begin using their children as a way to get drugs when they become old enough to be prescribed pain killers. Today's doctors will begin prescribing lose doses of hydrocodone as young as twelve and it sickens me to know that most of these kids are not even hurting but going in and lying to get their parents the drug. Missy was placed in this situation at a very young age and at the age of eight and a half she was getting pain killers prescribed to her for her Mother. When Missy was old enough to begin her menstrual cycle she was faced with Endometriosis a very painful conditioned and with this came the early onset of addiction for her. She would undergo surgery to remove one ovary and with *this and the pain from the Endometriosis she was using pain killers on a regular basis and began to use them as a pawn to get out of school. She would phone her Mother telling her she had pain killers and make a deal to give her Mother some in return for her getting out of school early. This was the family circle that has got to be broken, this type of parental behavior does nothing more than destroy the parent, child relationship as well as destroying any bond the parent had with the child. In Missy's case , she tried to go get help she took an ambulance from Moncks Corner to Downtown Charleston to get help from the local hospital, but unfortunately the hospital said there was nothing they could do, told her to go a couple of blocks up to the Charleston Center a place where they help drug addicts. At that moment Missy felt like no one cared, she was exhausted, dope sick, she was alone, and felt as if all the people around (which was medical staff) had their eyes on her, and on top of all of this she had on no shoes only sock, she never felt so orphaned and alone than in this moment. In Downtown, Charleston it is all concrete, in the summertime it is SO HOT. She walked the couple of blocks to the Charleston Center, where they said, "we are sorry, but we have no beds available for you yet, but we will have one in two days (Friday). Two employees walked Missy to another hospital, but once again there was nothing they could do. Well, when Missy left the hospital she had no way home, she asked the people walking by her if she could use their cell phones, and she tried to call anyone that could come get her, but no one did. When Missy was walking she saw a boy about her age sitting on a* park bench with an older man (you need to understand something Missy isn't your average white girl, God gave her a sense for people and she was smart) she was talking to the boy her age and they got up and started walking, the boy told her he wasn't going to leave her because they were downtown. Missy then, asked him, "if he did heroin", he said, "yeah I do, that's where I am going to now". Now this brings us to where Missy ended up on the streets of Charleston South Carolina's "East Side". The two of them walked into East Side, got the Heroin and they started walking back to where the boy said he lived. The young man told her, "I am a "street kid", " I live on the top floor of this parking garage". When they got to the top floor, Missy saw a piece of cardboard a pillow and a blanket, they sat there and snorted the Heroin. Missy loved it, and immediately wanted more The pair left the parking garage to get something to snack on, the boy taught Missy how to pan-handle (which she didn't like to much). They were at a gas station when a man driving a taxi wanted to know where to get some pills, and of course Missy knew, she made $60 off that deal. Missy seen someone standing around the gas station they tried to talk to her, she said she knew the boy who was five years older than her. Missy had the man in the taxi take her and U (the guy's name) to his aunt's house which was located in section eight housing. When they arrived they got out, and Missy asked him if he knew where to get any Heroin from he told her, "yeah girl, but you have to wait until daylight", they went and sat on his grandparents porch at about 2:00 a.m. Since it was the end of July it was hot.

When 7:00 a.m. came around the two of them walked to the corner store, there was people outside, and on some days the crack addicts would be saying, "where the dope man at I need my rock before I go to work". U found her some Heroin "boy" and they started to walk. living in abandoned houses and trap houses as a heroin addict at the age of twenty. Missy is lucky that she is still alive today to tell her story. I have seen women much older and much wiser than this young woman end up lying in an alley way dead in these same areas in which Missy lived homeless. God was definitely this child's Saving Grace, he placed many earthly angels around her young and fragile body to protect and keep her safe during the days in which she was lost, wandering around trying only to survive just one more day, one more fix just to get her through until she could get into a facility to get clean. Missy has told me many stories of her days as a heroin addict and my heart swells to the point I feel it will burst for if she had been my daughter I would have walked every street and searched every alleyway until I found my precious daughter even if she were an addict she was a daughter first and even before that she was the Lord's little angel whom he placed in the arms of her Mother to protect and provide for her. There are now days when I take her in my arms and hug her tightly because I want her to know just how much she is loved. Upon first meeting Missy it was a somewhat memorable event to say the least, standing in line at the outpatient clinic, I listened as an apparently tormented young woman no older than my youngest child Rachel who is 20 years old, lash out at the young man who was standing behind her. In a loud and almost violent manner she was screaming at this young man about something to do with the male species not understanding anything when it came to the female thought process. She shrieks out in a glass shattering voice that would remind most of us on a good day of a Jewish Mother from Jersey squealing out at her children on an episode of Sapranos or something and it was all I could do not to laugh at loud, yet cry out for her at the same time because I knew what she was doing I had done it all myself many times because this was the only way she could say what she wanted, when she wanted, without being told to shut up or screamed at by her boyfriend or husband I wasn't quite sure who he was that day but I would come to befriend the both of them as the days passed and I would grow to love Missy as if she were my own child. Listening to her and watching her moods I came to realize very early in our friendship that this was a young woman who was hurting so desperately inside that it would not have surprised me if she had exploded like a bomb at any minute. As time went by I began to talk to Missy and she began to confide in me about her past as I did her also in hopes that a part of my failures and grief's would somehow help this young woman who when I hugged her felt like a porcelain doll that if I held her to tightly would shatter all over the pavement. As our friendship grew I began to talk to Missy about God very early on, I don't remember how it all came about but I do remember the tears streaming out of the eyes of this woman as if she hadn't cried in years. Missy was so remorseful for her time into the world of addiction that she *thought God was angry with her, I explained to her that he wasn't angry but he was hurt, he hurt because just as any parent should his child was hurting. The little girl he had placed here on this earth and in the arms of a woman he hoped would choose a different path in life due to her own free will had instead created a young woman so strong, yet at this moment so frail because she needed someone to help her to understand what it all meant. Why did God allow her to fall into the pit of the Serpents Sting? Why had he allowed her to suffer the agonizing days of sickness due to the affliction of her drug abuse? I explained to her how much God truly loved her and how when she cried out for his forgiveness he was right there at that exact moment and she was forgiven at that moment, and the reason she continued to be burdened was because she had to forgive herself. Due to God not interfering with her freewill a woman of strength had been created, a woman with a voice as big as any leader I had ever met and as strong as any minister I had ever heard preach a sermon on Sunday morning. I honestly believe this young woman is on her way to becoming an advocate for women of addiction and for children affected by addicted parents. God knew that by letting Missy suffer the consequences of her actions that it would in turn make her strong and a survivor. With all the rage and anger that I saw being released in the early days of our friendship, I also began to see the love of Christ as we sat on the sidewalk in the wee hours of the morning and began a Bible Study that would help Mary grow at such a rapid pace in both her faith and her spirituality. As she began to soak in the Word of God* she began to calm and instead of lashing out in anger I began to see her acting out in love and kindness. Mary had a heart so full of love that she had placed on the back burner of her soul for such a long time due to the hurt she had suffered for so long. She felt as though no one really cared about Mary but what she didn't realize was how much Mary actually loved everyone. If there was anything she could do to help you she was there, but if you were not willing to help yourself she would get very agitated at your weakness and inability to stand firm, that was another issue she would have to learn to accept in some people. There are those of us who are so remorseful for the things we have done in becoming addicts and then there are others who are so lost and swept up in their addiction and loss of self-worth that they do not care who they hurt, what they do to their loved ones or the repercussions of their actions but what we forget is that when the addiction becomes so strong that it takes over total control of one's ability to think rationally, many people will get hurt. They say these types of people must hit rock bottom and sometimes rock bottom is death. Mary is a young woman and as she grows in age, maturity, wisdom, spirituality and sobriety she will understand these types of people more and more and she will see that iy was not the person a majority of the time but it was the addiction and evil that created that person who seemed so selfish and uncaring that they would jeopardize everything and everyone just to get what they wanted and needed, and we would end up on our road to recovery meeting many of these personalities on our journey. I pray daily for Mary and the young *man who she loves so deeply and compassionately. She would tread the fires of hell to save him, she would take a bullet to the head before she would ever allow anyone to hurt him and at this point in their relationship I sit back and watch as she desperately holds on with every fiber of her being. I want to say sweetheart back up and just be patient, allow this young man to also grow for he is battling the same demons we all are and to help her to see that if this relationship is truly in God's plan for her that nothing or no one can tear it apart but the two of them. They can choose to let the little things that do not matter go and blow into the wind for as I have explained to her the male mind is not like ours. They may be raging lunatics one moment and the next forget what they even were angry about, this is why they must let their relationship be based on the things of the upmost importance, love, affection, understanding, patience and most importantly, God.*

I have met many people since beginning my outpatient treatment. Some people have successfully finished the program while others have made several attempts only to find themselves falling once again into the grasp of the Serpent. Many people have died due to thinking they were in control and believing they could continue the methadone treatment while continuing to combine illicit drug use. Methadone is a very powerful drug used to treat both addiction and chronic pain but when used in combination with many other drugs it is fatal. Addicts need to be completely honest with their counselors and therapist about their drug use. There is always the possibility of slipping due to triggers which seem to occur a lot at the beginning of treatment but when you follow the program and keep the lines of communication open with the network created to help you achieve sobriety you can prevail. Addiction is vicious, ruthless and it knows no mercy, it will take a perfectly healthy body and mind and destroy them if at all possible, we must be willing to remember that we did not become addicts overnight so we will not achieve sobriety instantly. It is a slow process that will occur when you decide that you are not going to let the Serpent control your life any longer. When you make the decision to stop and place God in the center of it all, I promise you that every day in which you grow closer to Him and in the Spirit the closer you come to the day when addiction will be only a memory in which you can share with those who are suffering the nightmare which you once lived. When you take your accomplishments and begin helping others who have fallen victim to the cycle of addiction, you will not only be helping them but you will be keeping yourself safe by remembering through their pain and suffering what you once experienced and this will help you to continue the fight. This is a lifelong battle that must be taken seriously and as heavenly sisters and brothers we must join together to help one another conquer this affliction through God's Amazing Grace. He will continue to give use the power to overcome as long as we continue to allow him to be a part of our everyday lives and our everyday decisions. We must love one another and not judge because in the world of addiction, not one addict is better than another. We all have our demons which we battle every day and in reality all any of us want is for the hurt and the pain to go away, so when we stay strong in God's Word and

His Love there is nothing that will prevent not one of use from achieving our goal, SOBRIETY..

My Addiction, My Treatment

Sitting in my third grade class room awaiting my turn to give my essay on, "What I want to be when I grow up" definitely wasn't a drug addict. Little did I know at that age, an age when a natural high was the only life we knew as children that I would be faced with one of the most tragic forms of addiction known to mankind. The journey and long road to my addiction started at a very young age due to many childhood illnesses that only caused an inevitable path of being prescribed very potent pain killers that over a period of time and continued use would ultimately lead to a twenty year battle into the world of prescription addiction. Opiates, which are widely used today for anything from acute to chronic pain are one of the most addictive medications I have ever used and if doctors truly know the potential for this addiction they should be forbidden to prescribe these pain killers to anyone other than those who are suffering from severe pain caused from car accidents, terminal illness, and complex surgeries that would require only a short usage of any of these drugs. They say that anyone in chronic pain such as a terminally ill person cannot get addicted to these drugs and they are right because that person is probably going to die anyway unless a miracle takes place which would leave them fighting to recover from another deadly disease "The Addiction to the Pain Killers". Physicians must step up and monitor the dispensing of these lethal medications, especially the doctors who prescribe them for extended periods of time. The innocent victims who had no idea just exactly how addiction takes place or how dangerous the continuous ingestion of these pain killers really are until it is too late! BAM! It happens when you least expect it. You are sitting alone on the sofa and walk to the medicine cabinet to take a pill but realize there are none. The first day may not be so bad all according to just how many pills you take a day and how strong the doses are 5, 10, 30, 100mg. The higher the milligram the more severe the with draw. For a beginning user the actual cycle time to with draw is approximately 72 hours. During this time the person will experience, fatigue, sweats, fever, severe leg cramp and pain, stomach cramps, diarreag,
.

I began treatment at the out-patient program at the Center for Behavioral Health in fall of 2008. The treatment program I chose with the advice of my counselor was Methadone. I began with a dose of 30mg. and after a week went up to 60mg. It had helped me tremendously by taking away that terrible craving my body had always had for the prescription opiate morphine and morphine derivatives. For several months I stayed at the 60 mg. dosage but it wasn't enough to help with the excruciating pain that engulfed my body making it impossible for me to return to work and to have any quality of life. I later went up to a dose of 120mg. and after three years of working the program I returned to work. It was the first time in over 15 years I had been able to hold down a job without the consumption of massive quantities of pain killers. I truly wish that I could say that one day I will be able to stop using the Methadone but with the medical condition I have now and unless medical science develops a new way without the use of pain killers to treat severe pain I do not see it happening in the near future however, I truly believe Methadone was my saving grace, for had it not been for the Methadone Clinic and the many counselors I have had the opportunity of having to help me through the program I know without a doubt I would more than likely be dead now. I am not happy that I have to rely on this program to survive because sometimes I feel like I am just substituting one drug with another and for the most part I am but this type of pain management is completely different than all the others from before. I take Methadone and only Methadone for the pain. I now feel I have a purpose in life and I have some quality of life where before I lay in bed for days at a time drug sick because I had eaten all the pain pills I had been prescribed in less than a week. I do not recommend that anyone who is not truly ready to seek treatment begin this type of treatment program because I have watched as they come here only to get high, they use the methadone but then leave the clinic and go out and continue to use all the other drugs without thinking about the consequences. This drug is very dangerous and when mixed with other drugs such as benzodiazepams which will shut down the respitory system and stop the heart. Addicts are sick and deceiving and will use whatever means necessary to get their next high so it saddens me to hear when someone has died due to this disease. Addiction is a disease just like cancer, it is terminal and if it doesn't get you from accidental overdose it will eventually kill you by shutting down your system whether it be your heart, your lungs, your liver, your kidneys, or all of them in combination. Just like alcohol, long time abuse of opiates will lead to liver disease hepatitis and cirrohsis. As I stated in the beginning none of us ever said when I grow up I want to become a drug addict but today we can say I want to become sober, I want to beat this addiction that is slowly killing me and " I Want To Live" Sobriety does not happen overnight, just think of how long it took you to get where you are today but there is this promise every day that you continue with your treatment plan you are one day closer to sobriety and for now it is all about you. Take this time to work to become the third grader who once stood before the class and said " When I grow up I want to Be a Dr. Lawyer, Farmer, Fireman, Mommy, Teacher" whatever it is that you want to become the time is now and you can become anything your heart desires because my friend, It is all up to you.

    For me the Methadone Treatment Facility has helped me to continue on with my life. I hope that five years down the road I will be able to say I am free of any medication needed for pain but until that day I will continue to use this treatment plan because for now it works for me. I know that if the time ever comes and I am no longer able to pay for this treatment I will be forced to go back into the same hellish battle as I did before when I went through the withdraws from the other pain killers but for now I cannot dwell on that but instead work to keep my body as healthy and strong as possible so that if that day does come I will be able to fight it with a vengeance with the Lord God standing by my side I know I will be alright.I have the greatest form of ammunition the fight this war and it is Christ Almighty, he has given me the strength and the courage to make this journey one tiny step at a time and I realized, We don't become addicts overnight, addiction is a process that takes over so secretly, slowly creeping up on you until it has you within its selfish grasp, so, you cannot recover overnight either. Recovery is also a slow and painful process but please believe me that withdraws when they are over are nothing like the suffering you have faced as an addict. I promise you that sobriety will come and you will feel reborn. Once the poison from the Serpents Sting has been driven out of your body you will find it inconceivable that you ever became an addict. God Bless each of you who have taken or are about to take the journey, I will see you on the other side...

By: Letitia G. Carter

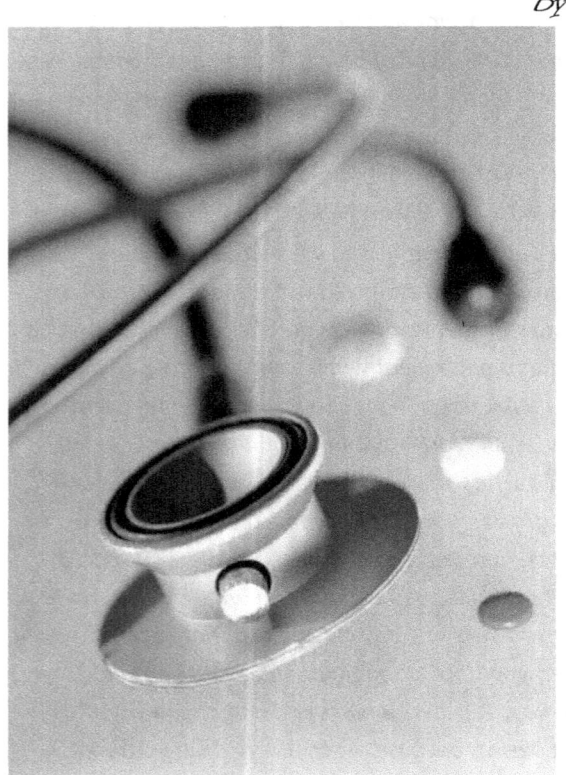

PRESCIPTION ADDICTION KILLS!!!

A Day Will Come

I sit back and think of all the beautiful days that I missed during my travels into the darkness of the Serpents

Sting. The trials and tribulations I suffered during my journey up to the gates of my Hell on earth. The pain I caused my children and all of those who loved me and I am so stricken with a sadness that will always be within my heart. Even though my children have forgiven me I know that neither of them will ever forget those days of darkness, it was as if a total eclipse had covered the sun and our world became as dark as night. My daughter went on trying to live as normal a life as she possibly could always telling me it was alright but it wasn't alright and I have excepted the fact that someday she is going to have to release that anger and that hurt in order to completely forgive me of my actions during those days when my addiction had peaked and I was left with nowhere to go but up. If I had ever wanted anything more in my life it was to be a good Mother, Grandmother, wife and child of God. My son too, is going to have to find a way to let go of his hurt and his anger in order to begin building his own life. I only want to take this moment to tell anyone reading this story whether you are a teenager who is curious, or a parent or child of and addict or someone who has suffered as my family and friends have suffered through similar evil forces of darkness such as my family has suffered, you are not alone. I have included a list of Help Crisis Centers that can help connect you with the right network of people who can help you begin the healing process. To each of you, May this next year be fruitful, may you accomplish more than you could possibly have imagined and may your strength and courage in the Lord Jesus Christ be the Light at the end of your tunnel. Peace, Love, and Joy to all…..

www.ingramcontent.com/pod-product-compliance
Lightning Source LLC
Chambersburg PA
CBHW080002210526
45167CB00026B/3806